Past Praise for Francine Falk-Allen's
Not A Poster Child: Living Well with a Disability—A Memoir

❋ 2019 Living Now Book Awards Gold Medal
Winner in Inspirational/Memoir (Female)

❋ 2018 Sarton Women's Book Awards
Silver Medal/Finalist in Memoir

❋ *Kirkus Reviews*' Best Books of 2018

"Overall, this is a frank, no-nonsense account of living with a disability, edged with a razor-sharp wit . . . Bold, charming, and inspirational."
—*KIRKUS REVIEWS*

"It's refreshing to see a sense of humor that leans absurdist rather than self-deprecating, and Falk-Allen's cheekiness enlightens as much as it endears. *Not a Poster Child* is enlivened by its uniquely compassionate approach to living with a disability as it confronts timely issues of vaccination, workplace accessibility, and life-affirming kindness."
—*CLARION/FOREWORD REVIEWS*

"*Not a Poster Child* places the reader inside the body of Polio—and into a world of surprising expectations. The view from Francine Falk-Allen's captivating memoir envelopes unexpected family dynamics and intimate insights only a writer who has 'lived the life' can bring to the page. As the daughter of a Polio victim, this book brought me closer to my mother's experience and into a reality few have walked..."
—PAMELA LIVINGSTON, MA, MFA, Book Passage

"With plainspoken eloquence, Francine Falk-Allen brings to life the rich palette of emotions of her lifelong battles with polio—the sorrows and joys, the heartbreaks and triumphs. Her book is funny, inspiring, and bitingly honest. It's a revealing, constantly surprising story that shines a new light on that eternal human question: how can we make the most of our lives?"
—EDWARD GRAY, Emmy Award-winning documentary producer and director

"A beautifully written book about loss, pain and finding the will to forge ahead. Falk-Allen writes openly and courageously as she details a childhood spent overcoming first, a bout with polio, and then [another heartbreaking loss]. With equal parts humor and irreverence, she takes the journey through young adulthood and finally to the current challenge of dealing with the late effects of polio. A first-rate memoir on all accounts."
—BRIAN TIBURZI, Executive Director, Post-Polio Health International

"*Not a Poster Child* is a memoir of wit, unstinting honesty and compassion about Falk-Allen, who contracted polio as a child and has lived her life as handicapped, and ordinary. But this is not an ordinary story. You grow to love this character who is our heroine... a story of a woman with disabilities which fade as she confronts the essential questions of how to make a life . . . with love and rejection, searching and finding, failure and success . . . unwavering in her willingness to take on life and make it work on her behalf. In the end the reader—this reader—has a friend and confidant."

—SUSAN RICHARD SHREVE, author of *Warm Springs: Traces of a Childhood at FDR's Polio Haven*

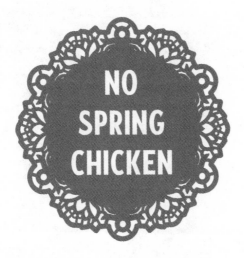

NO
SPRING
CHICKEN

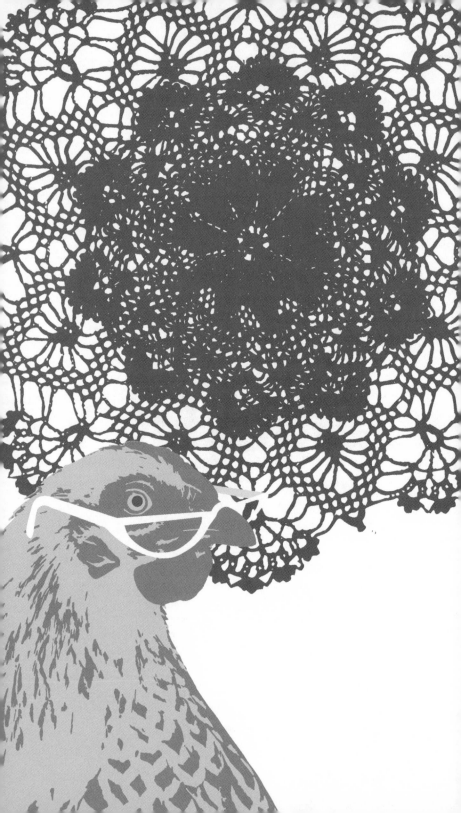

NO
Stories and Advice from
SPRING
a Wild Handicapper on
CHICKEN
Aging and Disability

FRANCINE FALK-ALLEN

SHE WRITES PRESS

Published 2021
Printed in the United States of America
Print ISBN: 978-1-64742-120-5
E-ISBN: 978-1-64742-121-2
Library of Congress Control Number: 2021900691

For information, address:
She Writes Press
1569 Solano Ave #546
Berkeley, CA 94707

Interior pencil illustrations by Francine Falk-Allen
Interior design by Tabitha Lahr

She Writes Press is a division of SparkPoint Studio, LLC.

For my nieces, Kathe and Carol

CONTENTS

———∘∘◇∘∘———

❋ Part III: Participating in Community

Introduction

————∘∘◯◯◯∘∘————

This is meant to be a companion book. Its sister is *Not a Poster Child: Living Well with a Disability—A Memoir*, the story of my life with polio and its after-effects.

A caveat, up front: Some people with disabilities do not like to be referred to as "handicapped," and I fully respect that. During the disability rights movement, the description "a person with a disability" became the preferred term—a social preference I was unaware of, even as a person with a lifelong disability, until 2018. I have almost always used the term "handicapped" to describe myself, because it denotes being capable but needing an allowance for a less-than-normal condition. So, my apologies if anyone is offended by the use of "handicapped." You do have to ask people with physical challenges what term they prefer, because it's not the same for everyone, just as a physically "normal" person might prefer particular descriptive terms.

Also . . . I thought a "Wild Handicapper" sounded more fun and kind of amusing, like an adventurous, untamed bird, and "Wild Disabler". . . well, it just didn't have a ring to it. I, along with most of the other disabled folks I know, don't want to be thought of as not having any flights of fancy left in me. Some folks with disabilities or who are simply aging are pretty feisty, too, often because they've had to be in order to get through difficult circumstances. So throughout this book, I will refer to myself and the person in your life to whom the material I'm covering applies (perhaps it's you!) as Wild Handicappers.

I contracted polio when I was barely three years old, in 1951, in Los Angeles, California. I was hospitalized for six months at a rehab facility for polio kids and adults (although I did not know there were adults there until a few years ago) in Santa Monica. We thirty or so children were confined mostly to one immense room the entire time we were there. It wasn't fun, but I got some interesting stories out of it (which you can read in *Not a Poster Child*).

I emerged from the hospital with a permanently paralyzed foot, and a mostly paralyzed leg that tried its best to grow but of course never became the full-length, muscled, functional leg that the other one has been. As a young adult, I felt robbed of my childhood in some ways, since I had to be responsible for my well-being from the time I was released, at three and a half, with crutches and a brace—new devices that I had to learn how to operate on my own. Later—in the 1960s, after becoming temporarily rid of the brace and crutches—I was kind of a wild child, as many of my friends were. I needed to re-grow up in my thirties.

These experiences shaped me not only physically but also emotionally and psychologically. It was difficult and yet, simultaneously, often irrelevant that I was a handicapped girl, and then a handicapped woman. A lot of my interactions with people and my other experiences did not happen to the average American child or woman, yet much of my life reads like just another baby boomer's.

In these pages are more stories about being disabled, especially regarding travel, and some things I've learned that you may find useful (or even humorous) if you have a permanent or temporary disability, or if someone in your life is handicapped or aging and you'd like to learn more about how to be with him or her. I don't claim to represent all handicapped people, but I know how it is for me, and I know how it is for a lot of "crips" I've met. (Within the handicapped or disabled community, some of us cheekily refer to ourselves as "crips," short for "crippled." This isn't popular with all disabled people but, as an in-crowd thing, it's not uncommon. Two things I have noticed are that disabled people tend to be really innovative about ways to deal with limitations, and they also often have an ironic or slightly absurd sense of humor.)

With regard to any suggestion I give, please check with your doctor or health practitioner before you follow any of my advice. My way may or may not be the best path for you. In any case, you are responsible for your results, and I hope they bring you joy.

I wrote *No Spring Chicken* prior to the COVID-19 pandemic, so I offer it up with the hope that we'll all be traveling and gathering again, clucking away happily, by the time you read this.

I hope you will find this book to be of value, and that you will share it with others. And do have fun with it.

— *Francine Falk-Allen*

Just Another Wild Handicapper

PART 1:

The Wild Handicapper Flies the Coop

Travelin' Girl

————o○○○o————

*A*s a young teenager in the early sixties—once I found out that I was a Sagittarius, according to western astrology—I used to like to get those little horoscope tubes you'd see at checkout stands. They were nearly always the same, but I liked putting myself into an interesting category and identifying with the attributes. Some horoscopes seemed to be quite accurate, particularly the ones about Sagittarians being honest and outspoken, their comments hitting the mark like an archer—and consequently needing to learn how to temper this trait, and be more tactful.

But most interesting to me was learning that, in this system, all Sagittarians loved to travel. I'd had little opportunity for that sort of thing in my short life. There had been one trip through Texas, Kansas, Utah, and Wyoming with my parents when I was six, visiting their birthplaces, the Alamo, and the Mormon temple in Salt Lake City (only from the outside); and then I attended successive summer camps starting between third and fourth grade. There had also been the blessed occasional week in Santa Cruz with my childhood friend, Daralyn, and her mom and little brother. But all of that had been no more than a taste or a teaser, and I wanted more—and due to the lure of the horoscopes, I now believed it was my natural right as a Sagittarius to travel as much as I could. (It was convenient to pick the traits I favored in this mystical system.)

Acquiring my first car, a brand-new 1969 Ford Econoline, at age twenty-one, allowed me the freedom I craved, even though the miles I accrued on the van were primarily in Northern California. I drove to my hometown, Yuba City, in the Sacramento Valley, first from San Jose State University and then, when I transferred to California College of Arts and Crafts for a year, from Oakland. Then, having moved north to Sonoma County, I drove a lot, because every town in the area seemed to be at least seven miles from every other town. Most of the roads were country roads, and I had friends all over the county— so, when my first husband and I argued, I'd drive down to Santa Cruz or up to Yuba City to visit friends for a long weekend, or go camping alone in Mendocino, just to regain some peace. All of this was easy, especially since I was in my twenties and had a lot of energy, compared to myself now (a woman in her early seventies).

Following in this and the next chapter are some overview bits about how I managed to adapt to driving with a disability, a little smorgasbord of what I've learned about general adaptations that are helpful when traveling, things to research when planning a trip, and the many benefits of travel (even when physically challenged), plus comparison of different types of travel, such as road trips versus air travel. And soon we'll get into fun stories about specific locales I've visited, with great success (or not). So settle back in a comfy chair and get ready for a good time . . . and keep your suitcase handy!

A Little Background

As a teenager and thereafter, I had to drive crossing my left leg in front of my right and sitting a little bit sideways and using my left foot for both the accelerator and the brake, since my right leg is mostly paralyzed and my foot is entirely paralyzed. (Well, I can imperceptibly move a couple of toes. I wrote about my futile efforts to improve that in my first book. Motor nerve damage is permanent.)

I have never had any ankle motion in my right foot, so forget pressing it down on an accelerator. I was only able to use my right foot in that way if I pushed from way up in the hip, which was extremely tiring and provided almost no control. (My crossover method cannot be done in a car with a very low steering shaft, so some rental cars have never been possible for me to drive at all; plus, hitting one's knee on the shaft over and over is pretty distracting, and bruising. I tried driving stick shift in Daralyn's car in my teens, pushing my right foot on the accelerator from the hip. It was scary for both of us and proved unrealistic even out on the many straight country roads in the Central Valley's flat Sutter County. So, I have never owned a car that was not automatic.)

After I met my second (and current) husband, Richard, on New Year's Eve, 1992, we began a sixty-mile commuter relationship of five years—ridin' on the "Freeway of Love," as Aretha sang. Driving with my left foot crossed over on those long, frequent drives started to give me back pain, so I quickly decided to get a left-foot accelerator installed in my car, which also was my first vehicle with cruise control.

The Magic of the Adaptive Accelerator

You can't just show up at your local mechanic's shop to get an adaptive accelerator. In fact, there are perhaps two places in the San Francisco Bay Area that install left-foot accelerator pedals. This is a relatively simple operation, but it can take a few hours, due to the placement of the mounting bolts under the chassis. The installation includes the addition of an apparatus inside on the floorboard that transfers the acceleration action from the usual right side accelerator pedal to the driver's left side with the implementation of a connecting bar. Conveniently, the interior device is easily removable—I can practically do it with one hand, and I'm a weakling—so even after installation, other people can drive the car without having to learn to drive "left-footed."

This pedal adaptation, though perhaps seemingly dry in its description, has been a liberating experience. Hybrid vehicles such as the one I drive currently present more issues for installation, but even with them it can be done.

I wish I had known about this adaptation when I was younger. Having it sooner might have saved some wear and tear on my now-arthritic back and allowed me to drive more and farther as a young adult. I knew there were hand controls for people who were paraplegic, and there may also have been left-foot pedal arrangements way back in the late 1960s, when I learned to drive, but I had not heard of this possibility or I would have looked into it.

The combination of an adapted accelerator and cruise control makes it possible for me to drive for longer than a half-hour without pain. However, I still cannot drive more than about ninety minutes per day without tendon pain repercussions and extreme fatigue, now that I'm older.

Making Travel Work for You

I did not let my polio-affected leg keep me from moving on out into the world, but serious travel has always been challenging, and is only more so as I age. That said, here's where I've been in the last sixty-five or so years. In the US, I've visited Hawaii, Washington, Oregon, Nevada, Idaho, Montana, Wyoming, Utah, Colorado, Texas, Kansas, Missouri, New Mexico, Arizona, Louisiana, Illinois, Georgia, Tennessee, South Carolina, Washington DC, Delaware, New Hampshire, Massachusetts, Maine, and New York. Whew. Internationally, I've been to Canada, Mexico, Pakistan, India, Egypt, Dubai (only the airport, let's be honest), Israel, the former Yugoslavia (or, on today's map, Bosnia and Herzegovina, Croatia and Slovenia), Italy, France, Germany, Switzerland, the Netherlands, Scotland, England, and Ireland. Yes, Europe and the Far and Middle East, cobblestones and all.

Many of these places were exceptionally difficult for me. When I was younger, I just assumed I could do anything. Now I am a lot more realistic—partly because I need to make things easier for myself, and partly because I am slightly wiser. I also used to be able to walk a mile or more as long as I had my cane. I'd be tired at the end, but I could do it. Now I need to stop and rest every block (or, more often, every half-block). I don't plan to walk more than about a quarter of a mile total on any day. (I did recently buy an electric fold-up tricycle, however, and it has made travel a fun experience again; you'll be hearing more about it later.)

What this difficulty means, for physically challenged people, is that we have probably three obvious approaches to consider if we really want to travel, assuming a lack of exceptional wealth:

1. *Make sure we have enough money set aside* to be able to take buses or cabs, tip all the porters, and stay in places that have elevators and no stairs. Travel is really not fun if it exhausts us to the point of having to spend every other day in bed. Taking fewer trips that are comfortable is more rewarding than taking lots of exhausting ones.

2. *Do a lot of advance planning*—which is probably going to be necessary anyway—to find discount trips, coupons, locations that are accessible, and places where it's just easier to get around.

3. *Accept the invitation of an amiable person* who offers to take you on a trip and either pay or make

things easier for you by helping out physically, or doing both. Hopefully you're lucky enough to have someone like this in your life.

If you want to travel as a Wild Handicapper, it's going to be more of a hassle if you don't try these approaches, and then you might find yourself thinking traveling isn't worth it—either after you arrive home, or even during the trip itself. What a shame that would be! So I suggest planning ahead and enjoying yourself.

Pack Light

My first airplane trip was in the late 1970s, when I went to Southern California for a meditation camp. On the way, I planned to visit old friends and stay with them, so I brought a variety of clothing—camping and go-out-to-dinner clothes—as well as a sleeping bag and a broad-brimmed hat. This is not an easy way to go when walking with a cane, because you can only use one hand to carry anything. In those days, rolling luggage was just beginning to show up (at least as far as I knew), and I did not have any. So I was carrying a big, lightweight, soft-sided suitcase and these other items. I sometimes had to carry the bag to a spot, put it down, then go back and get the sleeping bag, carry it to the suitcase, and so on. By the time I got through the first leg of my trip, I was already planning, with each limpy step, how my next trip was going to be better organized and easier. I was determined not to give up on air travel.

Soon after that trip, I bought a folding luggage cart, and later a rolling suitcase with a leash on it (which was like pulling a quiet but barely manageable big dog), and—later still—roll-aboard-style suitcases. I can't imagine being disabled in the 1940s and '50s, and carrying those big, heavy Samsonite cases!

I have never been great at traveling light and still am not. But these days, I use luggage carts in airports, or my darling husband schleps the bags or gets the cart, or I get a porter and tip him. It's worth it. (If you use an airport wheelchair, which I'll discuss later, the attendant will also expect a tip.)

In defense of my packing issues, I do have to bring along a considerable number of medically related items, including tapes for my tendon issues, a few pairs of adapted shoes, exercise bands, shoe inserts, medications, and a yoga mat (I trimmed mine down so that it rolls up and fits in my roll-aboard). I bring a gel ice pack—the kind that goes in a freezer—for my back and knee pain. Also, I bring a lightweight foam-rubber bathtub safety mat I bought at Target (and then cut down to two squares of about 18 inches each), paraphernalia related to my ankle-foot orthotic support brace, swim equipment for my pool therapy, sturdy sandals . . . The list of items goes on. It's difficult for me to go anyplace with just one suitcase, particularly one small one.

I have a girlfriend who travels to Europe from time to time and takes only one small roll-aboard that can go on the plane with her. This, for a three-week trip. She takes one pair of underpants and washes them each night, and one black knit non-wrinkle dress. She varies her ensemble with jewelry or a scarf, one or two pairs of pants plus tops, and two pairs of shoes—one walking, one dressy. Throw in some shampoo and makeup, and she's good to go.

I find this admirable, and also unfathomable; I realized I must be "high maintenance" after she told me about her sparse packing. I like a change of outfit, and I don't want to wash lingerie by hand every night. When my husband and I travel for two weeks or more, we plan to do laundry only once. We always take too much, but we take about half as much as we used to twenty years ago (which was mostly my fault).

Do Your Homework

Before you pack, you've got to plan this trip. As I mentioned earlier, I find that the farther in advance I do this, the more I enjoy my travels, and the less expensive or disappointing the trip is. Being physically challenged does not lend itself well to spontaneity and surprises, but that doesn't mean you aren't going to have unexpected experiences, both wonderful and challenging, when you travel. You can use travel guides and highlight things you want and/or hope to do. (You're unlikely to get to do them all, so there lies the spontaneity!) And, of course, you'll want to leave space for the times when you decide to cancel that tour of a museum because it is just so great sitting in a lovely park listening to the local school kids play jazz or watching people go by.

There are some places that are easy for handicapped people to visit, some that are not as easy but still doable, and some that I would say, *eh, I'm not going to see that place in this lifetime.* (Positano, Italy, comes to mind: it's built on a cliff, with many, many, many stairs.) So, think first of a place or places you have always hoped to experience, or browse online or in magazines or travel guides. Then I suggest that you find out if any disabled or handicapped people you know have been there. Get online and look for accessible travel; there are sites that make suggestions (see my Resources page at the back of the book). Most European hotel sites say whether or not there is an elevator. American motels and European or American bed-and-breakfast venues (B&Bs) often do not have elevators, so that's a primary consideration and something most physically challenged people need to know. I like to go to a bookstore and browse and buy guides, some of which do mention accessibility. I particularly recommend those by Rough Guides, Lonely Planet, and Fodor's.

I suggest you start with a comprehensive, free online e-book guide compiled by Martin Heng, formerly of Lonely Planet (see Resources). It has tons of info and disabled travelers' suggestions. It is not available in print; you put it in your online cart, go through the checkout process, and then download it and either print it yourself or just read it on your computer. Lonely Planet has a few accessibility guides for specific cities, as well.

Bon Voyage

Now that it is getting a bit harder for me to travel, and because polio management requires us survivors to limit our walking unless we're in a pool (the water holds us up so it's less effort than on land), walking is something I try to do only for pleasure and not for transport, which means I am more careful about which locations I agree to visit. If I were in a wheelchair permanently, I know I would be narrowing my vistas even more. My TravelScoot mobility tricycle has opened my horizons considerably, since it is easy to use in airports and on surfaces other than gravel or multiple inclines (a steep downhill that also slants in the horizontal plane as well, for example), and it folds up for car transport.

Traveling can be quite expensive; however, nearly everyone—even those with limited funds—can travel, even if only to an accessible motel in a nice area for a weekend away. I encourage all who have the travel itch to pursue getting out and about, if possible. If ever anyone offers to take you somewhere and assist you with any difficulties, take the offer and do not refuse! Don't be proud about accepting help. Yes, it is definitely more trouble to go places when you have physical limitations, and there will probably be some bumps in the road. But when you are sitting on a beach listening to the ocean and watching kids play or gulls dive, or in the cool redwoods reading a book, or in a car in New England seeing the colorful autumn, the extra effort will have been worth it. I know that some are content to stay at home (I love being home, myself). But travel is not only a refreshing and revitalizing change from daily routine, it also expands minds and teaches us about other people and places—even if they are just fifty miles away from our usual domain. I have found that narrow-mindedness is sometimes only inexperience wearing a cloak of apprehension.

It's so beneficial to get out of one's daily environment and tasks. The stimulus of a new or outdoor setting can be renewing, especially for one who spends either a great deal of time indoors or in managing one's health.

If you cannot afford a vacation, find a way to get to a park. Take a book (visit your public library) or just sit and watch the people and birds. Get yourself a cuppa at some cute little café with a sidewalk table and tell yourself you may as well be in Europe. Nearly every town, city, and country abode I've ever visited has had at least one nice place to sit for a while and recharge.

If you live too far out of town to be able to independently get around, I hope you have at least three more options: to move to town, to watch some travel films on TV, or to go out on the porch with a cup of tea and daydream.

Although it requires more planning and adaptation for me than it does for most, I have found that travel has been one of the great joys of my life. That Sagittarius teenager I once was had dreams of seeing the world, and I'm glad that I've managed to realize them. That girl was determined not to let a paralyzed leg keep her home in an armchair (though that's now also a favorite place to be). I hope that my suggestions in this book will encourage you to travel, too!

The Wild Handicapper

at Large

---oo0oo---

*H*ere we go! The trip is planned; put on your hat, ask your companion to carry your bags to the car, and promise to stop and buy him or her a latte along the way, or grab your rolling luggage yourself and find a safe way to hoist it into the car, 'cause we're going for a ride.

Take Me for a Ride in Your Car, Car

Car trips can be really great. They are cheaper if you are on a budget, as many handicapped and/or older people are; gas is still cheaper per mile in an auto (especially a hybrid!) than the cost of a flight, or even a train. You see scenery close up, or at least closer than in an airplane, and you can stop and stretch if your back starts to bother you (as mine does).

When Richard and I do a car trip, we try to vary our driving time; one day we'll only spend two hours in the car and another we'll go longer, usually with a maximum of five. When we drive longer hours, we always stay at our destination for at least two or three nights. We tried doing a one-night-stand trip in the northeastern United States twenty-plus years ago: We drove about four to eight hours a day with only a couple of two-night stays. It was grueling! And we were much younger then. We had vastly underestimated the distances and the quality of the roads. We vowed to keep destinations limited and stay longer at each place from then on.

In a car, you can also more easily take any apparatus you might need, such as a walker, a folding wheelchair, or a foam mattress pad. Richard and I rarely leave home without a mattress pad when we travel by car directly from home. Too many hotels (or relatives' or friends' homes) have beds with mattresses that are too firm for a person with back and limb pain. (In recent years, though, most hotels have improved, offering pillow-top or memory-foam mattress pads.) I take both my crutches and my cane in the car, too (though I do that on airplanes as well). I also appreciate that there's room in a car for a blanket to lay out in a grassy spot for a picnic or for reading a book.

The drawback to car trips is the length of time you spend sitting, especially if you decide to venture far. If you are going more than a thousand miles, I'd advise taking a train or flying, if you can afford to do so (and if airplanes or trains are not a physical problem for you). Then, if you need a car at your destination, rent one there. You will not be as tired as if you had driven the whole way there, and fatigue can ruin a vacation.

If you live in a lovely area, you can take very satisfying short trips with limited driving time. When we lived south of San Francisco, we used to drive just twenty minutes to Half Moon Bay on the coast and rent a hotel room, and we felt like we'd flown to San Diego. It was good simply to get away from housework, our to-do lists, and our land line with its telemarketers and robo-calls: very refreshing, and all we had to do was throw some things in an overnight bag (and pay for the hotel, of course).

When I didn't have much money, and before I became a bit creaky, I used to go camping regularly, especially up in Mendocino County. Later, I camped at Yosemite with friends, a tradition that continued for thirty years. Now, camping is too much work for me; packing all the cooking equipment, prepping a couple of meals daily, cleaning the kitchen area and tent each day—these are activities that are too painful for my back and require more strength and energy than I currently possess, although I loved it while I was able to do it.

Be creative. If you really want to go someplace, don't let a disability keep you from vacationing. Again, do some research and find places that are easier for you. I don't recommend going the nomad route; seeing where you "feel like staying" while out on the road or the railway is for able-bodied "normies" (a term some disabled people use for non-disabled folks) and young people. Planning will ensure that you will enjoy your vacation instead of being fatigued or frustrated by a lack of accommodation, such as finding that there is no elevator in your hotel or landing in a place where there is no restaurant nearby.

Leavin' on a Jet Plane

Now that I use forearm crutches often, particularly when I need to walk more than about a half block, I have found that I can still take my cane when I go on an airplane. I put it in a soft-cloth, easily foldable case designed for architectural drawings (I at first looked for a quiver, but they are all too small); then I use a cross-body shoulder bag on one side—no other choice with crutches—and put the cane case on over my head on the other side, with the cane resting on my back. I look a bit like a bandolier with the two straps crossing the front of my body, but it functions perfectly: it's lightweight, and it's no impediment to walking with my crutches.

Airplanes present their own special set of limitations—limitations you must put up with in order to get to otherwise inaccessible parts of the world. When you make your flight reservations, most airlines (but not all) allow booking an airport-use wheelchair online, which may be necessary unless you have a scooter. If they don't have this online feature, you will need to call the airline after booking your flight and tell them you'll need a wheelchair from check-in to the boarding gate, at arrival gates, and perhaps also—if you have greater walking difficulty than I do—from the gate onto the airplane.

I had been using a wheelchair in airports since I was in my early fifties, when I finally admitted to myself that I cannot walk long distances without extreme fatigue. In the last few years, airlines' information requests have become more nuanced. They often ask if you cannot climb stairs at all, cannot walk at all, or can get up from a wheelchair and partially function. I always say I cannot climb stairs at all—though I can, with difficulty—because I've had such ghastly experiences at Heathrow in London and Charles de Gaulle airport at Orly, outside Paris, in the past (see Chapter 8 if you're curious). Very small planes almost always require climbing stairs; "puddle jumpers" or commuter flights, such as the planes from Edinburgh to Inverness or Cozumel to Cancun, and other flights are considered "short," so be sure to check whether any flight is on a small plane requiring you to use stairs.

Charles de Gaulle airport now has the wheelchair transport issues there somewhat under control. However, you cannot get a wheelchair to take you all the way to the train station next to the airport, though the attendant will tell you she can take you there—because she thinks a quarter- to a half-mile is "close," and that's how far away from the train station they have to drop you off. If you cannot walk at least a quarter mile and do not have your own scooter or electric wheelchair, you should exit the terminal and take a taxi to the train station.

Thankfully, Heathrow has been remodeled since some mishaps I had there, but do tell the attendant if you cannot climb stairs so he or she can plan the route through the airport. The last time we had a connecting flight there, it was easy. The attendant took good care of us—thank goodness, since it was a very long walk (at least a mile) that I could not have managed. There was even a reasonably good pub in the airport where we had a nice lunch. However, if I could avoid Heathrow, I would, unless the cost were otherwise prohibitive. It is one of the main landing and connecting airports from the US when you are traveling to continental Europe, so you might not be able to bypass it. If you can, though, take a direct flight to Stansted airport in the north of London; it's much smaller and easier to navigate, as may be Birmingham in the west of England. If you're going very far north in England, Edinburgh airport in Scotland is also small, fairly efficient, and easy to navigate. There's also an airport at Newcastle that has limited international flights in and out.

Some airlines still put all the wheelchair people in one area of the plane and insist that they wait till every single last straggling, half-asleep normie passenger on the plane disembarks. If this is the case, you'll hear an announcement prior to landing saying that those needing assistance getting off the plane or those anticipating wheelchairs should wait "until all other passengers disembark." I think this is a product of our societal unwillingness to wait an extra minute or two for anything, let alone a handicapped person trying to crutch or cane his way off a plane.

For those who need a wheeled transfer chair, it is imperative to wait, but if you have a short connecting flight or train to catch, you'd better tell the chief flight attendant and hope that they are sympathetic. (My recommendation is not to have connecting flight intervals of less than ninety minutes, ever.) And if you can walk, even on crutches, get yourself together as quickly as you can and disembark with the other passengers. They aren't walking much, if any, faster than you likely can, with all their gear and kids, down those narrow aisles. This insurrection may cause you to have to call for a wheelchair at the gate and wait for it, unless there's one waiting for you, but you'll at least be off the plane and on your way about a half hour sooner.

Some airlines assume that if you need a wheelchair to get to the plane, you cannot walk at all. (France in particular is sometimes a bit snobby about handicaps.) However, an organization based in Paris, *la Caisse nationale de solidarité pour l'autonomie*, or CNSA (The National Fund of Solidarity for Autonomy), assists the handicapped with various issues. Perhaps most useful is the Parisian English-language site AngloInfo (see Resources). You may be able to check there for updates about current expectations and requirements.

Boats (*Les Bateaux*, "lay bat-OH") and Trains (*et les Trens*, "eh lay treh")

(Hope you enjoyed the French lesson there.)

I've taken long train trips in the US, and they were fun for the first few hours, especially when it was light, because western states offer such amazing scenery. You can explore the train a bit, get something to eat or drink, read, and have a conversation with your companion or someone you meet. But if I ever again rode a train for more than six or eight hours, I'd get a sleeping car. I arrived exhausted when I took the train from Oakland, California, to Montrose, Colorado (eighteen hours to Salt Lake City, UT, and another few hours to Montrose, changing trains once or twice), and also from Oakland to Portland, Oregon (fifteen hours).

In Europe, unless we are only staying someplace one night because we have a layover, we always plan to stay in each city or town several nights, as with our American car trips. It is really tiring to keep packing up and leaving each day. If you want to see the countryside of France, you could take one of those canal barge trips, but you do need to be able to get off and on a small boat easily. If you are in a wheelchair permanently, this won't be advisable for you unless someone can lift you on and off and help you around the boat. A river cruise on a larger boat or the Mediterranean can usually accommodate a wheelchair. On a boat cruise, you don't have to unpack and pack over and over, but sometimes these trips are tightly scheduled, with a lot of early rising.

Our canal trip in the south of France was quite lovely, but one of the boats in our flotilla of two was too large to go up the Grand Canal, so we partly motored along the Mediterranean, viewing the dumped old boats and other industrial debris and having thoughts that this had not been our vision of a canal trip. We decided to joke about the absurdity. Eventually, we went up another canal, and it was scenic, bucolic, and lovely. There were places we could not dock with the bigger boat, so in those cases the barge personnel came and got us in a van and ferried us from village to village. This was not as convenient and relaxing as docking in a town and just climbing off the boat for a look around, which is what most canal trips with smaller boats offer. Since I did not yet have my electric tricycle, the ancient towns with their cobblestones were difficult for me (larger cities tend to have flat sidewalks, maybe because of women's high heels?) and would be prohibitive for someone in a wheelchair unless it had large wheels and possibly shock absorbers. It was still a good trip; fantastic food and the company of friends made it memorable. But if you do something similar, I strongly recommend that you book a boat that can go up the Grand Canal, and that you prepare yourself for a lot of tricky walking in the little towns.

If you are not on a boat trip, I suggest planning to go to no more than three cities during a given European trip, unless you'll be there at least two weeks. For able-bodied people who walk a great deal, this would not be necessary, but for a handicapped person, it's the smart way to go. The trains are really comfortable and run frequently in Europe, and they're a good way to get from city to city. And I've begun to see portable ramps provided in some stations (all the stations in the United Kingdom have them). Still, getting luggage, a wheelchair, a walker, and/or a large scooter, plus yourself with a cane or crutches, on and off a train can be cumbersome. There's often a gap between the platform and the train, plus one or two steps to negotiate.

We actually had a very easy time of taking the train in Scotland, Ireland, and England in the summer of 2016; in those countries, they provide luggage, equipment, and boarding assistance for the handicapped if you call or email ahead—and sometimes even if you don't give advance notice; the station staff almost always offered to help.

If you are going to travel by train, either take a few small pieces of luggage or travel with someone who will lift your larger bags on and off the train for you. In India, there are porters who will handle your luggage for a few rupees per bag, but in most of Europe today, porters are not seen as often as they once were. If you are affluent and are taking the Orient Express, perhaps your luggage will be handled for you! (That's a dream trip of mine . . . Maybe someday.) I have not seen people in wheelchairs on European trains, ever. I believe this is changing as countries try to make train travel accessible for people of all abilities. During a UK trip in 2016, I did see U-rings on trains for clipping security straps to a wheelchair or scooter, as have been common in the US, where there is generally more accommodation for handicapped people.

In the States, if you use crutches or a cane, I find that there is often a willing American ready to lend a hand. This is not so true in Europe, for the most part. There are kind, thoughtful, helpful people everywhere, of course, but in my experience, the US, Canada, the UK, and Ireland are the places they're most likely to offer a seat on a crowded train or bus, open a door, or voluntarily extend other types of assistance. I wonder if handicapped people in other countries stay home a lot more than we do here. There may be an assumption in other countries that there are things you just don't get to do as a handicapped person, and places you just don't get to see, and that you should know that. But I also think it's partly that people outside the US are more hesitant to intrude on others' lives, even to be helpful. It may be that Europeans feel they should not embarrass you by asking if you need help. Here in the States, we have little inhibition about approaching others, for better or worse. In general, Americans seem to be more willing to get involved in other people's lives by offering help. (To be clear, this observation does not refer to all Europeans; I simply have had more people offer help in the US.)

Country Girl Goes City

I have found that most American cities are a great place to take a vacation. Walking issues are minimal because you can usually get a cab to just about any place you want or take public transport. Richard and I don't rent cars in large cities with good transportation; we only rent them to get out of the city to other destinations. For instance, as much as I thought I might not like New York City, because it's so crowded and New Yorkers have a reputation for being rude (at least in laid-back California), I was astounded to find that I loved NYC. There is so much to do and see, and my experience was that the people are not very rude at all; in fact, they are for the most part quite friendly. (Driving in that city, however, is the worst in the world, other than in Cairo, Egypt.)

When Richard and I go to NYC, we usually stay near Times Square, because we always see at least one show and the theater district is so close. If we get stuck and cannot get a cab, a Lyft, or an Uber, it's only about three blocks back from any theater to our hotel—a distance I can walk if I have to, as long as I stop and rest every block. Also, the larger hotels there sometimes have a pool where I can work out the kinks I get from sitting on an airplane or sleeping in a bed that is not optimally comfortable. (When we stayed in Paris for two weeks once, we shopped not for perfume but for an "egg carton" foam mattress pad; it was well worth the expense. That hotel—our favorite, Parc St. Severin in the Latin Quarter—now has more comfortable mattresses. We may have made a point with them. Oh, and if you stay there, tell them we sent you; they are lovely people and will take great care of you.)

One drawback with NYC is that if you go someplace a bit out of the way, you may end up stuck for a while until you can get a car to pick you up. This can be a problem if you cannot stand up for very long, or if it's raining. If you do not have a smartphone, when you leave your hotel, make sure you have the number of a good cab company. The bellman or the concierge will be able to tell you the best taxi to call if you are unable to get a Lyft or Uber. (When we travel internationally, we get foreign service activated on our mobile phones and make sure we have the hotel's number when we go out.) A few times, we've had to call our hotel and ask them to call a cab to come get us. Keep in mind that if you do this, you'll be charged an extra fee, since the taxi driver is going out of his way to pick you up. But on the plus side, the cabbie also knows that when he gets to the hotel he'll likely pick up another fare, so he'll be quick about picking you up at the far-flung restaurant, museum, park, or other venue where you've found yourself stuck.

I don't use subways anywhere anymore because there are always too many stairs involved. Even the ones that have escalators don't always have them in places where you need them, particularly up to the street, that last leg always being a long flight, and you often have to walk a block or two (or more) underground to get to your transfer train. I used them in NYC, Paris, Barcelona, London, and Washington DC before finally coming to the realization that they were wearing me out. It's more expensive to take cabs or ride-shares, but we budget that into our travel expense. (And now I have my folding electric tricycle for closer destinations.)

Buses are a great way to see a new city, but you need to get a bus system map (and make sure you know enough of the language) to get around. Taxi drivers almost universally speak at least a small amount of English—enough to understand where you need to go—which may or may not be true with Lyft or Uber drivers; we have had some in foreign countries who spoke no English. Cabbies transport to and from hotels a lot, and deal with a lot of tourists. You can also have your destination(s) written on a slip of paper. But don't count on a bus driver in a non-English-speaking country speaking English, since his passengers are mostly locals. You may want to at least know how to say, "Which stop?" in the local language and have the destination written out, and hopefully the driver will tell you. Of course, you have to get on and off the bus, and this may not be an easy proposition, depending on your physical limitations. In the US, many cities have buses with wheelchair lifts (San Francisco and Berkeley have them, for example). That's another thing you will need to find out before you book your travel, if you are planning to use buses. Contact the local transit agency at your destination(s).

Getting What You Want—and Need

Please don't be daunted by the research you need to do. This is all in the interest of having fun. Once you get it all squared away, it will be mostly smooth sailing. And, in the process, you will learn things about where you're going. You may find you want to stay at one place or another longer than you'd initially thought, and you may want to skip another place that is going to be difficult or has only one aspect of interest to you. For instance, if you're handicapped or traveling with a handicapped person, resist that suggestion that you "just have to see Positano, Italy." It's a hillside city known for its beauty and views, but (as I mentioned previously) it's full of stairs and steep roads and paths. I'm glad my husband saw it before we met, and if you are really curious, it's featured in a number of videos about Italy. Sometimes being an armchair traveler is enough. Comfy chair—and low cost, too.

Whenever I book a hotel, I try to get a place with a swimming pool. My first priority is no stairs (so mostly no bed-and-breakfasts, unless they have rooms on the same floor as the entry and kitchen). My second is having a restaurant either in or near the hotel (i.e., not more than two doors away), and my third is a pool. If I have a lot of options, I will even call to see what the pool water temp is! I also always email that I cannot be lodged more than two or three doors from the elevator (I have ended up at the end of very long hallways where I had to stop and rest every few doors, an exhausting experience). I also let the hotelier know that I need a quiet room because I am such a light sleeper (due to polio discomfort), so they don't put me right next door to a noisy elevator or vending machines.

In the US, if these requests get mixed up or ignored, and I do not get a room that accommodates my handicap, I ask for a generous discount or room upgrade. In other countries, I sometimes ask if there is something they can do "to make it right," and occasionally I will get a room upgrade. In foreign countries, the concept of "making it up to someone" is not as prevalent, I've found, but you can always try. You may be met with a shrug or insistence that the situation could not be helped, but you won't know until you ask . . . politely. The other thing to remember in foreign countries is that Americans singularly tend to have an attitude of entitlement that is not common elsewhere, other than among aristocrats. (I'll tell you a story about American traveler attitudes in a moment.)

The Americans with Disabilities Act (the ADA, passed in 1990) requires accommodating disabled people if advance notice is given. This should not be narrowly interpreted as simply putting you in an ADA room (which is always nearest the elevator). I always email or call to make sure the hotel understands this when I make my reservation, and generally carry with me a copy of the request—and the response, if I get one via email. I call the hotel a day before arrival and make sure that I am going to get what I asked for. If they say at that late date or upon arrival that they no longer have a close room, I assert myself, ask to talk to a manager if necessary, and explain that I requested this because I am handicapped. Hotel managers are generally very accommodating about this, probably because they do not want to get involved in any discrimination issues, especially with the ADA in place.

I always ask *not* to be put in an ADA room. They are very good for people in wheelchairs, or those who need a roll-in shower. But if you are not in a wheelchair or using a walker, these rooms generally have smaller, lower closets with a low clothes pole (not good for long dresses or coats, and I never wear short dresses because I am self-conscious when my orthotic brace shows), less furniture, and fewer amenities, such as a loveseat or an easy chair (less furniture allows more room for wheelchair turnaround). ADA rooms almost never have bathtubs, either; instead, they do have roll-in showers with a seat—which often have slippery floors. Just be aware of what you are going to get and make sure it's what you want. If you say you are handicapped, they almost always put you in an ADA room, unless you ask very specifically for a standard, non-ADA room (in a similar location, if you need that).

Okay, here's the story about American attitudes.

I traveled in India and the Middle East with my English friend Patricia Epps (and several others, all Americans) for three months in 1982. Some of the men on our trip were demanding of waitstaff, and it sometimes embarrassed us women. While we were discussing their behavior, Patty told me, "When I was a waitress in England, I hated waiting on the Yanks. They wanted their beer cold"—England often drinks it room-temp—"and their food hot, and they wanted it now. I always thought, 'What cheeky bastards.' Then I came to the States, and I understood why they were so pushy. You can get your beer cold, your food hot, and get it now. Yanks are used to getting what they want and so aren't afraid to ask for it." She gave me a wry smirk. "Now *I* want my beer cold and my food hot, and I want it now!"

Yes, there are other countries with bad manners, too. But that doesn't mean we Americans can be pushy in other locales and expect other cultures to make allowances for *our* bad manners. As ambassadors of an affluent and innovative country long known for inviting the tired and hungry masses with open arms (until the Trump era, at least), I feel we should be on our best behavior and consider what we want other countries to think of us. It's always preferable to make friends rather than offend, right?

That said, I've been pretty dang annoyed a few times with unaccommodating hotels after I've originally asked nicely. They have sometimes heard directly what I thought about their performance. But I think the most effective thing to do after working to get your needs met and having been disappointed is to write an honest review on a site like TripAdvisor. If I have either a very positive or very negative experience regarding my disability, I use "Great for handicapped (or disabilities)" or "Terrible for handicapped" as a review title. And, of course, tip the front desk staff appropriately if they helped you, or at least give a hearty thank-you at the time and again upon leaving.

All European cities have their challenges, but many are surmountable and worth meeting. Yes, there are cobblestones—but, as I've said, in the major cities the sidewalks are usually flat and easily negotiated if you are walking. If you are in a wheelchair or using a scooter, it will need some terrain-friendly wheels, because you will have to go off the sidewalk from time to time. Using a walker will not be as much of a problem, if you're already used to negotiating curbs and lifting it when you need to.

Paris, France, and Edinburgh, Scotland, are my favorite cities in the world (so far), but I also love New York, Seattle, Vancouver, Canada, and of course San Francisco (that one is only lower on my list because of the difficulty of those famous and picturesque, but very steep, hills).

Un Petit Journeé á Paris

These days in Paris, at many corners and at many doorways, there are ramped entrances, although some small shop entrances have only token ramps that are very steep and short and would require someone pushing from behind or pulling you up backwards to manage them in a wheelchair. In the late 1990s and early 2000s, I saw almost no ramped entrances there. The last time I was in Paris, I even saw an electric wheelchair in the Latin Quarter. Next time I go (and I hope to), I'll take my motorized trike. If I had not bought it, I'd have planned to look into seated scooter rentals.

The first time I went to Paris, I was ill-prepared, but fortunately I was able to walk for longer periods in those days (I was thirty-five). Even then, going to the Louvre was extremely tiring, as was negotiating the long walks between Métro stops and the stairs up to the streets.

Ten years later, this time traveling with my fiancé, I knew what I was getting into. We still mostly used the

Métro, but this time I looked at all the hotels we were considering on maps before we booked so I knew we'd be staying as close as possible to a Métro stop. If you are still able to do stairs without much hassle, I recommend staying within a block or so of a Métro stop—which will likely be good for the rest of your party, too, disabled or not.

"Taxi!"

Another wise move is to stay in a hotel near a taxi stand. You might not have this figured out before going, but if you think you may revisit the same city, be sure to mentally note which hotels are either very popular (all the taxis will come there frequently) or even take actual notes on where the taxi stands are. Taxis, in Paris particularly, often only pick up fares at taxi stands. They are regulated in most cities, and city governments don't want taxis stopping to pick passengers up at random, especially on one-way streets, since it interferes with the flow of traffic. Our favorite hotel in Paris has a taxi stand about one block away, which works fairly well for us. If I'm wearing dressy shoes for the evening, we have the concierge call us a cab— or we do it ourselves, especially now that we use Lyft—to meet us at the hotel. There are sometimes designated areas for Uber and Lyft, although in cities they tend to pick up just about anywhere; hotels sometimes still give preference to taxis, though. (Again, be sure to get roaming or foreign service on your mobile phone, especially if you plan to utilize this form of transport on your trip; or, alternately, you can use a SIM card for specific countries, or a temporary phone, while you're out of the US.)

How Near, How Far?

One warm summer day in Paris, we asked our hotel concierge, Benoit, how far it was to a particular restaurant, Le Petit Prince de Paris—a place we'd heard had excellent food and a fun atmosphere. We had about fifteen minutes to get there.

"Ah, *oui*, it's not far," Benoit said. "It will take you about five minutes."

Thankful for the generous time frame, we set off, me with my cane and Richard with his boundless energy. Twenty minutes later, after walking several blocks and hiking up a moderate hill, we still were not there yet, and I was nearly exhausted. We realized that for Benoit, this was a five-minute walk, but it was about a half mile, which for me, with my taking a break to lean against a lamppost or sit down in a sidewalk café every block or so, is at least a half-hour's walk.

Ever since that experience, if a clerk at the airport, a concierge at a hotel, a storekeeper, or anyone else I'd expect to be able to estimate distance accurately tells me, "It's very close," I ask how long it takes to walk it, and then at least triple the time. I sometimes ask, "How many blocks?" because most people cannot estimate distances very accurately, and asking, "Is it a quarter-mile?" will usually get you an answer of, "Oh, no, it's not that far." When I hear their time estimate—which, in European or city terms, is for an able-bodied person who not only walks everywhere very quickly every day, but also carries groceries home in both arms—I know whether I can do it.

People will often look at me with my crutches or cane and still not understand that a block is far enough, two is pushing it, and beyond that may be a hardship or necessitate allowing twenty minutes to include stops for rest, or even require a car ride. On a leisurely day when Richard and I plan to stop every block or so and sit down, it's less of a problem. People don't understand walking limitations unless they have had them; even nurses and doctors who deal with these problems on a daily basis often don't translate their knowledge into practical circumstances. (Exception: My polio doctor! She totally gets it.)

Whenever someone tells you, "It's close," it's wise to be skeptical, unless it is very easy for you to walk a mile or more. I don't look decrepit, so I get a lot of bad advice. Be prepared to get a lot of that in Europe, where everyone walks everywhere at a pace unseen in California. (This is why they get to eat pastries all the time, and we don't.)

Challenges aside, Paris is a fantastic city overflowing with art, history, and music. Classical concerts at St. Chappelle near Notre Dame are etheric and life-affirming; we love also the medieval art and music offered at *Musée de Moyen Age*—the "Museum of the Middle Ages"—and the cellar jazz clubs, with their jazz *manouche* (the non-slang term for gypsy or Django Reinhardt jazz). We're captivated by the gorgeous parks of Paris, and the often-great food. It's a feast for the eyes just to ride around in a cab. We feel at home in the Latin Quarter, which is near a lot of sights we like to revisit (you can walk only three or four blocks in any direction and have a full week of art, shopping, eating, and music). It's full of little cafés, some of which have remarkably good food and some of which are good enough, but all of which are easily navigated; since this is the university area, there are many students working in the shops and cafés, and they all speak English willingly. Our favorite hotel, Parc St. Severin, is a half-block from Rue de la Harpe which is lined with cafés, one of which is a *crêperie*. Yum. And connected to that street, toward the Seine, is rue de la Huchette, with several little jazz cellars.

The first time Richard and I went to Paris together, we took a tourist bus around the city for an hour or so and got an idea of which places we'd like to spend more time visiting. This is a smart and pleasant orientation step if you will only be there for a very few days. (The same goes for Barcelona, and I would imagine the same to be true for many other big cities as well.)

Bicycles and Scooters

If you are able to ride bikes (and like to ride them), the rental bike stations that have been cropping up all over the place over the last few years are another great option. If I could ride one, I'd certainly do so. You rent the bike with either Euro coins or a credit card, and when you've finished your ride, leave it at the nearest bike stand and go on your merry way. Pretty cool! Not for me, unfortunately, but some handicapped people can ride bikes.

I rented a scooter twice in Dusseldorf, Germany, when my husband's former company sent him there. That is a great flat city for a seated scooter, if you stay in the downtown area. I was all over the place! They have some remarkable architecture and museums accessible by taxi, as well.

Mini electric scooters (the kind that one rides standing, like a skateboard) are available for rental in many cities now, but not all the issues about how and where they can be left have been worked out. In San Francisco, some have been thrown into the bay by San Francisco natives when they've found them left strewn across the sidewalk by renters who seem to think that's okay. I'm unable to use these, but if my issue were simply fatigue and not paralysis, I'd use one (with some caution) for short distances. I think they look like fun, and I have a little envy for those who can take advantage of them!

Now you have a bit of an overview of ways to get around in cities. I hope that, armed as you are with this information, you are looking forward to booking a hotel in some new, exciting metropolis.

North, South, East,
West—US and Mexico

ou don't have to venture across the Atlantic to have a great trip, that's for sure. Here are some of the places I've been in and near the US, and some helpful info about what is easy or difficult about them for the physically challenged traveler.

San Francisco

San Francisco is a somewhat difficult city for those with a walking problem, much as I love it. It has so many steep hills. But there's so much to see and do, and Golden Gate Park is so lovely. There are wheelchairs at all the museums. American Conservatory Theater (ACT) and Sydney Goldstein Theater (formerly the Nourse) are a bit difficult: no elevators. But generally, when we go to the city (it's just over the bridge for us, a half-hour or so from our home), Richard drops me off very close to our destination, and then finds parking. Sometimes, when I feel less fatigued, I walk to the garage with him afterward; otherwise, he gets the car and picks me up. I have had friends do this favor for me as well, but it's important to remind them that dropping me off and picking me up will take extra time.

Once, an especially valiant girlfriend pushed me all the way up the spiral ramp at the Academy of Sciences; I will not have anyone do that for me again unless I lose half my weight, which would probably mean I was dying. My husband, meanwhile, has missed the beginning of some concerts in order to take care of my drop-off and the parking. I always feel guilty when this happens, but in my defense, he's often late on his own as well. Birds of a feather.

Mexico

I used to go to Mexico somewhat frequently. I've been to Barra de Navidad, Guadalajara, Mar de Jade, Club Med at Playa Blanca, Puerta Vallarta, and Cabo San Lucas in Baja California. Mexico is generally a less expensive place to find a resort, but even the prettiest places south of the border are sometimes less than functional. You might have to be prepared for an uneven trip hazard in the gorgeous tile floors, or questionable plumbing, or doors that don't lock, or construction going on next door to your supposedly pristinely quiet suite or condo. Some areas also have a high crime rate, so just check with the US State Department before making your reservation, and don't drive anywhere at night.

In some places in Mexico, you can eat vegetables without fear, while in some places you cannot, unless they are cooked. So, no salads (hard for a Californian). Avocados, onions, and cooked meats and fish are usually okay, however.

If you speak Spanish (mine is extremely minimal), notify your hotel in an email or fax, or by phone, what your specific needs are, such as no stairs. Most higher-end resorts have personnel who speak English, but even then, a staff member wishing to be polite on the phone may say they understand what you are requesting when they actually do not. It's a good idea to at least look up the words so you can get the idea across. The Mexican people I've encountered have generally been really great about trying to meet me halfway on vocabulary and communication. For instance, I tell them I have a "*mal pie,*" a bad foot; I try to explain that polio caused it, so they understand that it is not just a stubbed toe; I say it is "*dificil para mi caminar*"—difficult for me to walk. (I looked up "bad foot" recently, and the real translation is "*pie lesionado,*" meaning "injured foot" or "foot with a lesion." That's clearly not quite accurate in my case, and it seems that they've been getting my meaning with "*mal pie,*" however, so I may just stick with that.)

If you are easy-going, you can have a very nice time in Mexico. In the best-case scenario, you'll enjoy the relaxing and slow atmosphere, get a respectable tan, eat some delicious Mexican food, drink a little sangria or tequila, and meet some very amiable people. Of course, the crime factor has been exacerbated by the malicious activity of violent drug lords in much of Central America in recent years; Mexico is slowly trying to eradicate these issues but hasn't succeeded yet. For this reason, we have not been down there for a few years.

The Southwest US

As we leave Mexico, I'd like to give a quick nod to the Southwest US. Albuquerque, Santa Fe, and Taos, New Mexico, are definitely worth a trip. You will find excellent museums and art galleries, great food, and the opportunity to learn more about Native American culture. Tucson, Sedona, Scottsdale, and Phoenix, Arizona, are also an easy set of warm cities to visit—mostly flat, always a bonus! Richard and I also love the beauty and culture of Boulder, Colorado.

Aloha, Hawaii!

Hawaii is a particularly easy, warm, and restful destination. I've been repeatedly, to a total of four of the islands. It's a great place to get some rest with a nice balance of a little activity. For a US destination, it's not cheap. Because of its geographical isolation, many things have to be shipped over there, and since it is primarily a tourist destination, they even charge more than you'd expect for things that grow there. Remember that any place where real estate is at a premium (Hawaii is made up of islands, after all), rent costs more and property taxes are higher, so those costs get passed on to the consumer. But you don't have to adapt to a different currency, they speak English, and it's tropical. That's a lot to offer.

Unless you plan to park yourself for the entire time at a resort or other destination that is going to transport you to and from an airport, you really do need to rent a car on the islands. This may be prohibitive to those who need adaptive vehicles, but if someone else can drive, you can work this out. (And given how many older people go to Hawaii, I'd advise contacting a few car rental agencies or medical equipment agencies; they may have an adaptive vehicle.) I have always spent considerable time driving or riding in a car when I've gone to Hawaii, because there's very little public transportation (that I've noticed) between areas. There may be tour buses, and there are public buses on every island, but I haven't seen them often. And while the fact that most of the towns and cities on the islands are small in comparison to other parts of the US—the tourist destinations, at least—is a plus in terms of them being quiet and friendly, it's a minus regarding frequent public transport. I'm sure Waikiki has a lot of taxis, but I cannot recall ever using a taxi in Hawaii.

One caveat and caution regarding car rental in Hawaii: the last time we were there, in November 2017, we waited in line at the Maui airport for over a half hour to get on the car rental shuttle, and then, even though we had a reservation, were at the car rental lot for an hour waiting to get our car. Good thing it wasn't raining, because there was not an interior place to wait. I had never had this experience in any of the years I'd previously been to Hawaii, but it seems that something has changed, so bring some reading material in your carry-on. There may be some agencies that will allow you to pick up the keys at the airport and grab your car at the lot, or that are more efficient in other ways (we rented from Enterprise as we have on many occasions in many cities), but I'm not aware of them.

On Oahu, I especially do not recommend the lower-cost car rentals such as Dollar and Budget, because they are far away from the Waikiki airport. For a handicapped person, this is a hassle not worth the (possibly) lower price. You'll have to navigate getting to and boarding the shuttle with your luggage, a long ride, and possible long walks to get your car with these off-site rental cars. Because of this, I always rent from an agency that's close to the airport. But if you have plenty of time and energy, go ahead and save your nickel. (And actually, given what happened on Maui, perhaps there is no longer a way to save time when picking up a rental car in Hawaii!) Next time I go, I plan to carefully read the TripAdvisor and Yelp reviews of island car rental agencies before picking one.

Each island has a rainy side (normally the east, where it's jungle-y and lush), a desert-y side (the south), a windy side (north), and a side for lovely white beach sunsets (west). On all the islands but the big island of Hawaii, you can see virtually the entire island in one day if you get up early. That said, my feeling is that you shouldn't go to the Hawaiian Islands unless you can stay at least a week. It takes about three or four days to "get the mainland out of yourself" and really relax. Hawaii has a slower pace, so plan for enough time to enjoy it.

I'm going to go into some detail about the individual islands here, because for a handicapped person there is not an easier and more beautiful place to go to for a vacation. It's warm, so circulation is not as much of a problem as it can be for limbs that are atrophied or paralyzed. And no one expects you to do a lot of anything there, which can be an issue at other vacation destinations where busyness is considered getting the most out of a locale. (It is humid, especially in warmer months, so if you don't like that, I don't recommend going in the summer; that's why it's cheaper there from June through August.)

Anyway, here's my ode to the Hawaiian Islands.

Maui (Rhymes with Wowie)

Maui is my favorite Hawaiian island. It has not only all those beach and shore environments I mentioned above but also, in the middle of the island, an "upcountry" that's a lot like Sonoma County, California, in its appearance and country-living lifestyle. Maui is also the second-largest island of the chain, so there is a lot to do and see. If anyone in your party is antsy and bored by a lot of relaxation, there's plenty to amuse. There are large and little towns with their own identities, beaches with very different activities, a lot of windsurfing and regular surfing to watch in different areas on the north coast, and some snorkeling, too.

If the risk is worth it to you, I recommend going for a helicopter ride to see the island from overhead. I was squeamish about going, but it was a life experience I found awe-inspiring. There is no other way I would ever have seen any of those spectacular tropical valleys or remote cliffs, since I'm not capable of hiking in. So I researched which flight companies had the best safety records, resigned myself to a little fear, and got into the 'copter. It's true, whirlybirds are not as easy to control and land if they get into a pinch as planes are—and honestly, I didn't know just how dangerous they are when I took my own trip—but just sayin', much of the scenery took my breath away, and when we set down on the tarmac, I was sorry it was over. I felt euphoric, almost giddy, and privileged to have seen all that lush, remarkable beauty.

Taking a day to drive over to the Hana side of the island is a great way to see some lovely country. The road is quite winding and narrow most of the way, so it's a slow but exquisite journey. There are canyon parks along the drive where you can take easy, scenic walks; don't miss the grove of rainbow eucalyptus trees at marker 6.7, which have multicolored bark that looks like it's been painted in an array of colors—pretty psychedelic. Richard and I kept saying, "Wow, look at *this*!" There is also the Garden of Eden Arboretum at marker 10, which boasts more rainbow eucalyptus, along with a large variety of native plants, as well as a reasonable admission fee.

You may want to spend the night at Hana, which I would do if I went again, because it takes three or four hours to get there from the west side, and then you must turn around and drive back the way you came; you can't drive on the southern road that loops around back to the west, as it is a gravel road for most of the way and is really only for local traffic. The long drive is worth the scenery, in any case!

I have several favorite restaurants on Maui, including Mama's Fish House near Paia on the north coast, Ko at the Fairmont on Wailea, Ferraro's, the Italian terrace restaurant at the Four Seasons at Makena on the west coast (those three are all expensive "special evening" or "occasion" splurges), and Sansei, an amazing Japanese seafood place in Kihei (also on the west coast), an affordable spot where a lot of locals go for celebratory parties. But there are many more wonderful spots of varying prices, so do your research (I like TripAdvisor or advice from someone who either goes often or has been recently) and find your own favorite eateries and lodgings. You can get some good packages, too, if you keep an eye out for them.

For scooter rentals on Maui, I have used a place called Gammie's. They are reasonable: they rent by the week (some scooter rentals only offer a day rate), they allow some grace about your departure time, and they will deliver to your hotel and have a scooter there upon your arrival. If you are staying at a big resort, renting a scooter is a necessity if you have walking issues, and will make your trip far more relaxing and fun. I like to have a little energy left to go to a museum, take a walk in a botanical garden, or crutch my way down a charming shopping block. A scooter also comes in handy for getting around in shopping centers or even on a beach. Many Hawaiian beaches have a flat lawn area between the street and the sand, and paved walkways through the parks or along their perimeters. You can sometimes navigate from your hotel to a beach and only have to go a few steps into the sand to get the whole beach experience.

The Other Islands

Kauai is remarkably beautiful. It's probably best for a romantic getaway where you do not plan to do much, or if you want to go on a solitary retreat. There is supposed to be good snorkeling on the south side, and I would consider that area also for some really nice resorts—good for honeymooners, I've heard. Kauai has an area on the northwest side that is supposed to be spectacular for hiking as well, but I'll never see it except in pictures—unless I go on another helicopter ride. If you have someone with you who wants to hike while you read a book on the beach, it might be a good island for you.

The north shore of Kauai is full of condominiums, many for rent (somewhat like the west shore of Maui). It doesn't take long to get from one place to another by car, unlike on Maui or the big island. You can easily drive the entire island in a day—minus the west coast, which is almost all wilderness and bounded by cliffs.

The big island, Hawai'i, is huge in comparison to the others. It takes about three hours to drive east across the island coast to coast as the crow flies, from Kona to Hilo, on a road that is basically straight, through country that is mostly desert until you get to the east side. But that's what you do if you want to see Hilo (an area similar in appearance and weather to Maui's Hana), unless you fly into Hilo in the first place or pay extra to fly from Kona to Hilo. You also must drive if you want to see the volcanoes, which are clearly major attractions, although in 2018 they were erupting and spewing lava pretty seriously and visiting them was not just dangerous but actually impossible. Assuming that is not happening when you visit, I do recommend making the effort to go to Hilo; it is really a strange thing to step on warm volcanic rock, and it's arresting to see the devastation lava is capable of causing. I have only seen lava flowing into the ocean (near Hilo) in films, but that is quite spectacular, if you get the opportunity.

The Kona and Kahala (west) side is the most popular. It's quite desert-y but has some nice beaches, albeit not many white-sand ones. I hear there is very good snorkeling, too, which is often true of places that have warm water and lava rocks instead of fine sand. There are a lot of vacation time-share rentals in the area. I was lucky enough to stay in a lovely house near Kahala with a friend once, but I did need a seated scooter to get to the beach and the little local restaurant. Kahala is mostly residential, so you'll need a car to get out and see anything other than the local beach house, beach, and café. There are resorts at Kona which are quite nice, and you'll still need a car to go resort-, restaurant-, and sight-hopping.

Oahu is underrated; people immediately think of Waikiki, *Hawaii Five-O*, and Don Ho when they hear it mentioned, but if you get out of Waikiki it's lush, quiet and relaxing. Waikiki is a big city by Hawaiian standards and, though it has lots of things to do and see—great restaurants and the Bernice Pauahi Bishop Museum, for example—it's busy and crowded.

If you fly into Honolulu and are not flying on to a different island, get a rental car service that is located *at* the airport, as I mentioned earlier—and then I recommend heading to the eastern side of the island, where there are a lot of charming little towns and beaches (that side of Oahu happens to be where President Obama likes to go on vacation). It's very laid-back and pretty; I like to go there to paint. We rented an inexpensive house on a quiet beach when we went, and that was just the ticket. There's also a botanical garden you can hike through and up into the island, but of course I have not done that.

The north side of Oahu is awe-inspiringly beautiful, too. There are lots of little places to shop up there, and good surfing to watch up on the northeast side near Turtle Bay.

I have not been to Lanai. I always thought of it as the pineapple plantation island, but of course Dole pulled out and moved to the Philippines, leaving many Hawaiians with no jobs. I understand there are places there that you can rent for weddings and other gatherings—secluded spots hard to find on the busier islands.

Neither have I been to Molokai, which was known for its leper colony in earlier years. Now it is a quiet retreat destination; I've seen it from a helicopter, and it looks gorgeous.

The last and smallest island, Kahoolawe, off the southwest side of Maui, is too small and dry for any lodgings, but you can take a boat out that way to dive or snorkel at Molokini, a nearby crater reef.

Although I don't think I could live in Hawaii—I'd get island fever and miss the ability to drive a long way before encountering a beach, not to mention the cultural aspects of the San Francisco area—it's certainly one of my favorite places to visit. Easy, warm, beautiful scenery, relaxing, good food, mostly friendly people, and particularly accommodating for those of us with physical challenges: it's pretty hard to beat for a respite.

It's always hard to bid "Aloha" to Hawaii, but we'll have a great time in the national parks of the US—our next stop!

Getting Outdoors
in the USA

———⊶∘◦○◦∘⊷———

I need to get out in nature regularly. The refreshing green of just about any foliage (other than poison oak) at once calms and re-energizes me. But the natural world is often inaccessible to physically challenged folks.

The US National Park Service (a branch of the Department of the Interior) stated in 2012 that although there are few national parks that meet the NPS goal of "opening opportunities to people with disabilities," they want to improve this. Over $120 million would be required to repair national parks enough to make them all accessible, and some of the 419 parks have embarked upon this. Disability activists describe this upgrading as "an ongoing battle." The NPS also has come to realize—thanks to comments made to them by disabled travelers—that we want more than a boring one-mile stretch of pathway when we visit our national parks and crave more access to nature, and this doesn't have to mean over-paving wilderness areas.

According to an article from Roadtrippers.com and another from OutsideOnline.com (a branch of *Outside Magazine*), the most improved parks for handicapped access are Yellowstone National Park, in Idaho, Montana, and Wyoming; Staunton State Park, Colorado; the Grand Canyon National Park, Arizona; and the Statue of Liberty, New York. The best trails, according to Outside-Online.com, are in Acadia National Park, Maine; Grand Canyon National Park, Arizona; Glacier National Park, Montana; and Yellowstone National Park.

Having not been to those places before (I will be on a Utah national parks trip at the time this book is being edited), and also having run into pathways at state and national parks that start out well and then crumble into disrepair and become impassible, I can't speak for them all personally—but I can highly recommend Yosemite National Park in California.

Big Rocking Out—Yosemite

The majesty of Yosemite Valley in eastern central California beckons me nearly every summer. My husband and I make the long, winding drive from Marin County, across the Central Valley, and up into the hills and down again, to hang out with friends by the lazy Tuolomne River, surrounded by trees, and gaze at the valley's astounding glacier-cut granite. I have found that it's a very accommodating National Park for a person with a wheelchair, scooter, or even walking difficulty. There are even accessible places away from the crowds, though most of the trails adapted for wheelchairs or scooters are in the more populated areas. I've found that it's possible to reach many meadows and wooded sites and picnic grounds, the museum, the ancient graveyard, the Ansel Adams Gallery and gift shop, other shops and restaurants, and more— plus the Village Store for groceries or an ice cream—with very little difficulty!

Camping in Yosemite—for the Ambitious (or Cash-Strapped) DP Traveler

For twenty-five years, until I was about sixty-five, I "car camped" at Housekeeping Camp in Yosemite Valley, right on the riverbank, with a large group of friends every year. Richard joined me when I was in my forties, when we were dating. There, each unit has a tent with three concrete walls, beds with acceptable mattresses, a modestly furnished patio with a privacy fence, and minimal lighting and electricity. There's also a pit campfire for each unit, and you can bring your own Coleman stove and/or hot plate to use. Some of the units are accessible by wheelchair, but some have soft dirt that has to be traversed from the camp road, so if you cannot walk one hundred feet or so, ask for either a disabled person (DP) or ADA unit or a unit close to the road when you reserve, and be sure to say that you have a disability and must have this.

The shared restrooms throughout Housekeeping Camp have toilets and sinks (and are generally wheelchair accessible). It became too hard for me as I got into my sixties to pack all the gear needed, plus do the actual housekeeping required in camping—there's a reason it's called Housekeeping Camp—to keep doing the camping trip. But it's the most accommodating and comfortable place to camp in the Valley, though not a quiet wilderness or isolated camping spot.

There is one DP bathroom in Housekeeping that's equipped for wheelchair showers, with at least one accessible unit nearby that you can reserve. I can't recommend the shower, which when I used it was like having a warm water hose over your head (they may have fixed it by now), and the main Housekeeping Camp showers are not roll-in accessible. However, if you are staying in either Housekeeping or Curry Village, which is nearby—a reasonable scooter ride or quick car trip from Housekeeping—you can use the newer, more spacious, pleasant, and accessible showers at Curry. That area has a few accessible lodge rooms and cabins, and a lot of tent cabins, all with no cooking or campfires. Curry also includes a cafeteria and a few modest but acceptable cafés and food stands. Nearby are campgrounds where you can pitch your own tent or park an RV, and cooking is allowed in those camping areas.

If you camp in Housekeeping or Curry Village or the nearby campsites, or stay in Yosemite Lodge, you will need to reserve a year and a day in advance, unless you want to try your luck calling the reservation desk every day starting about a month before you want to go and cobble together a few nights in succession; there are always cancelations, but this is a labor-intensive process. (Please see my Resources section regarding the helpful National Parks Yosemite disability guide.)

If you were one of the old Yosemite devotees, like myself and my friends, who were disappointed in 2012 by the confusing change of many iconic and historic names for places in Yosemite, weep no more. Although the management company whose contract ended had copyrighted the names, the National Park Service finally won them back a couple of years ago—at a cost of $12 million! For those who visited Yosemite for the first time in 2015–2018, sorry, but the names you learned while you were there have reverted back to the originals—names that are familiar to millions of old campers and are now permanent. Those are the ones I'll use here.

Richard and I began staying at Yosemite Lodge in the Valley in 2012. It costs twice as much per night as Housekeeping Camp (in 2020, about $280 vs. about $110), but it's great to have a bathroom in your room, a lot of electrical outlets, and a better mattress. I don't miss traipsing to the communal toilets in the dark or using my makeshift arrangement in the tent, though I do miss waking up in a tent unit near our friends and sharing a quiet cuppa in the mornings. Each room in the Lodge has a private patio and also a mini-fridge, so we bring small coolers of dairy foods and fruit and prepare breakfast, and often lunch, in our room. Sometimes we walk across the street to the food court and eat with the tour group masses if we want a cooked breakfast, but honestly the food is . . . well, *meh*, for the most part. There is also a pool at the lodge that's often nearly empty in the mornings. The lifeguards are generous about letting me use float devices to do my water therapy, even though there is a rule against using them in the deep end. When I've explained to them that I am a polio patient, they've always kindly let me bend the rules. (The pool closes after Labor Day until Memorial Day weekend.)

It's nice to go to the Ahwanee Hotel at least once to view the outstanding early-twentieth-century Julia Morgan architecture—the Great Room and the Dining Room are lit by two-story windows and surrounded by tall, graceful trees—and have a drink or lunch on the patio. The breakfast buffet is expensive but pretty good, and there are awesome views through the two-story windows. For a special dinner, though, we prefer the Mountain Room at the Lodge, which does not require a jacket or tie and usually has at least one dish to satisfy a foodie. The Mountain Room also has a very good breakfast buffet, similar to the Ahwanee's and less expensive, so that's where we usually go for a big group brekkie.

Exploring the Valley

I recently started renting an electric sit-scooter in the Valley at the Lodge bike stand (they have only one or two, however). My TravelScoot is a little too lightweight for some of the bumpier trails or soft dirt, so I rent their larger scooters. Now I can smell the pines and see the butterflies and wildflowers up close. An especially great benefit has been that my husband and I are able to go a few places together without the car, with him either walking or riding his bike.

The park does its best to discourage car use in the Valley. The Valley shuttle, with its wheelchair lift and bike rack, is a helpful asset and goes nearly everywhere, but since I am not in a wheelchair, walking from the shuttle stops to my destinations is still too much. (The shuttle lift can handle scooters and power chairs up to 750 pounds, max size 24" x 46," and there are tie-downs inside the bus. I don't know if the scooters rented at the park exceed this size.) A walk from the shuttle stop to, for instance, the interior of Housekeeping Camp can be the equivalent of a couple of blocks to a quarter mile, which is a long trek on crutches. However, many of the shuttle stops are right in front of the place you want to be.

Specific and clear maps of the shuttle route are available throughout the Valley. They also show the safest routes for wheelchairs and scooters. I take the scooter from the Lodge over to Housekeeping Camp each day (twenty minutes by scooter and five by car). We take the car to the campsite for campfires in the evening and cook with the group. If you don't know someone who is camping, there are sometimes evening ranger campfires in the Valley, with entertaining historical presentations. There are also tours of the Valley floor that allow you to see it all at once fairly quickly, and perhaps determine which sites you'd like to revisit. From almost anywhere in the area, you can enjoy spectacular views of Half Dome.

Along the road to Mirror Lake (a dry lake overgrown by a meadow), you can drive a car in for a mile or two if you have a disabled person placard or license plates. I like to park and then walk about thirty feet to sit by the Tuolumne River and read, paint, chat, or just contemplate. If you have a motorized chair or sit scooter, you may want to scooter in a couple of miles, until the paved path at the end of Mirror Lake Road crosses the river.

A sometimes highly populated jaunt for a scooter is the one-mile paved trail up to Lower Yosemite Falls (across from Yosemite Lodge), an awe-inspiring view even in the summer, when there's less water falling. The trail is interesting on its own for anyone who likes geology or finds beauty in intimacy with rocks and trees, too. There is also a partially hidden spot off the main path (there's a sign that says something like VIEW POINT) with a perfect distant view of the falls where I like to go and sit for a while.

I've made it up to the foot of Bridal Veil Falls, which is nearly always still running in the summer, but it is a pretty steep trail. My husband pushed me in a wheelchair for the first portion, and I walked using my crutches the rest of the way. It's a pretty challenging walk, even for those with matching legs, and the Park Service warns of this to those with ambulatory or especially breathing difficulty, but there's a nice spot to sit once you're up there. Another thing we like to do is park across from the bottom of the mammoth cliff, El Capitan, and spot rock climbers with our binoculars. Careful you don't get a stiff neck; it sometimes takes a while to sight climbers who appear to be the size of toy soldiers hanging on the rock face!

About an hour northeast of the Valley, Tuolumne Meadows awaits those who want a little more peace and quiet in wide-open spaces. My husband and friends generally go hiking for a few hours, and I park myself somewhere near the river and paint a watercolor. There are a lot of places not far from the dirt and gravel access roads where you can feel somewhat isolated but still safe, if you don't mind using wilderness-style bathroom practices and are able to walk about one hundred feet from the road. Right by Tioga Road (Highway 120, which was originally a Native American footpath, then a Sierra Wagon road, and then a mining road), especially near the little general store, you'll probably see people every few minutes. But if you sit with your tunes and earplugs, you won't notice their conversations.

There are also lovely places to sit near the rushing Tuolumne River. When I have gone a quarter mile or more away from the highway (assuming I can find a parking space!), near Lembert Dome, Tuolumne Meadows Campground, or Tuolomne Meadows Lodge (a tent cabin site where you can purchase refreshments), I have seen hikers approximately every thirty minutes. A ranger usually leads a walk by there every hour or two as well, which gives me a feeling of someone responsible knowing where I am. At the same time, I get a bit of the isolation in nature that I crave and cannot achieve in the same way as those who can hike far into the hills.

Beyond the Meadows is Tioga Pass "Resort," a lodging of cabins and a café, and east of that is a long, steep drive down to the desert location of Mono Lake, the little town of Lee Vining, and Highway 395, the north-south road on the eastern side of the Sierras. At the Whoa Nellie Deli at the Mobil gas station on a hill above that intersection, you can get a very good meal, including a buffalo burger and some of the best chocolate cake you will ever experience. It's not hard to find, there is picnic seating, and lots of travelers avail themselves of the welcome repast and a place to sit and enjoy the view.

Back south of Yosemite Valley, about an hour's drive up from the Valley, is Glacier Point, which is a premier vista point. The very steep quarter-mile walk from the parking lot to the top of the path will allow you to view Half Dome at its same level, plus the entire Valley far below, and many of the surrounding granite peaks. I recommend a wheelchair or scooter unless you can take your time and rest repeatedly along the way. Remember that this is at very high altitude—7,214 feet above sea level—so you will be shorter of breath than you would be back down in the rest of California.

If you skip the eastern turnoff to Glacier Point and keep driving south a ways, an hour south of Yosemite Valley is an area called Wawona, which has the lovely old Wawona Hotel. The food is good and the rooms are mostly charming, though I am not certain it is completely accessible. Also in that area is Tenaya Lodge at Fish Camp, which is a real four-star resort with nice accommodations located in a lovely site. It's also a good place for a conference, large family gathering, or reunion. Both are not far from Mariposa Grove, home of the world's most ancient, awesome, and huge-girth trees, giant sequoias. The grove is well worth a half-day's visit. You can also go horseback riding in this area (a concession that is no longer available in the Valley).

I think Wawona would be a nice place to stay on the way out of Yosemite Valley if you're headed south. If you want to access the Valley and/or Tuolumne Meadows more than once, however, the drive is a bit too long and winding to make it a realistic overnight location; it would be at least a two-hour commute each day.

If You Go Down to the Woods . . .

During our 2014 trip to Yosemite, I scootered my way back from Housekeeping Camp to the lodge on the paved path around dusk, with hikers and bikers passing me occasionally. One couple I passed was walking right on the curb, dangerously close to the road, and I was tempted to caution them but decided to keep my own counsel.

While casually enjoying the woodsy scenery surrounding me, I saw off to my left in a little clearing a huge bear statue that hadn't been there the prior year. I was thinking it was a little odd that they'd put one in that particular location . . . when the statue turned its head and looked at me!

The (very much alive) dark brown bear was about six feet long, nose to tail, and three or four feet tall on all fours. Its head was a foot wide, including ears—the size of a grizzly, but there have only been black bear species in this area for decades (and they can be either brown or black in color). He or she was wearing a green collar placed by the park service, so he was clearly known in these parts; his territory; overwhelmingly not mine. He was a mere twenty feet off the path, watching me motoring by.

We stared at each other, our heads slowly moving in tandem, as I scooted past, and suddenly it seemed the scooter was not nearly fast enough. He took a step toward me, and as he (or she!) did I realized that ocular contact was absolutely the worst possible thing to share at that moment, so I tore my eyes away, adjusted the scooter to top speed—maybe 6 mph, a bit dangerous on the curvy, bumpy path—and began to think of what I was going to do if the bear followed me. Hmmm . . . start beeping the horn, since all wild animals hate and are intimidated by noise (though the horn was not loud enough to be optimally scary). Then maybe throw my backpack toward him, even though it had my laptop in it (with all my writing on it; I back my work up, but sometimes forget to do so). Bears know backpacks sometimes contain food, and I figured that was the most interesting aspect about me from a bear's perspective; after sunset is about the time animals are thinking of checking out campsites for unattended food.

Please, oh please, not my laptop; just turn around, Big Bear! I pleaded silently as I scootered away, and I kept looking over my shoulder every few seconds till I was sure he was not following me. Now I understood why that couple had been walking so close to the road!

After I'd gone about a quarter mile down the path, I was sure he was not in pursuit. A lumbering bear is easily heard from a distance; we'd heard them often enough in the middle of the night when we camped in Housekeeping. My heart rate had gone up during the encounter, but it had all happened too quickly for me to be very alarmed or upset, or even decide if I'd been courageous.

A few of my friends at Yosemite have had even closer and more direct encounters with bears, and no one's ever been attacked. The bear would win, so it's important to know how to behave with them. Normally, you slowly back away from these beasts, especially if it's a mama with cubs, but I hadn't had that option on this occasion.

The next afternoon, I nabbed a Mammoth Beer coaster at the Mountain Room Lounge at the Lodge, picturing the giant head of a bear that looked just like my new pal. I have it displayed in my kitchen to remind me of my good fortune, both in seeing the bear and in his disinterest in following a small human on an unfamiliar little vehicle.

The following year, I was conscientious about getting back to the Lodge before dusk. I found, though, that I was a little wistful at the bear's spot and scanned more deeply into the woods in that area each day, slightly hopeful I'd see him again.

Even if you don't engage with a bear, there's probably a deer, squirrel, or marmot waiting to meet you at Yosemite or one of the US's many other incredible national and state parks—so make your reservation!

Capital City and the Big Easy—
Plus Way Up North, Eh?

————◦◦◯◯◦◦————

*H*ere are a couple of other US destinations of which I am fond; I think you will find much to recommend them. Our nation's capital is not only the center of our government but also a cultural gem, and New Orleans is just plain fun! I include Canada at the end of this chapter, because, well, it feels like a sister country right next door, and is so easy to visit, either by plane or by car.

DC and New Orleans

New Orleans and Washington DC are two more places that are fairly handicap-friendly and well worth visiting. Both cities have acceptable taxi service (DC has a subway system but we found that we were still doing more walking than worked for me) and are full of things to see and do that do not involve walking long distances. Now, of course, I have my mobility tricycle, which made our last trip to New Orleans much easier. We look forward to descending upon DC again one of these years.

DC

DC has a lot of museums, many of which provide wheelchairs for onsite use, and great little jazz clubs and bistros out in Georgetown—mostly on or just off U Street, as I recall. We saw the aging Charlie Byrd play guitar in a small club not long before he joined the heavenly orchestra, and also saw Sonny Rollins play dynamite sax at Lincoln Center.

I had vertigo on the DuPont Circle subway escalator, which is two or three stories tall. I have acrophobia in very high places, such as on the Eiffel Tower or over a gorge, unless I look straight out; they give me the very real sensation that I'm about to fall—which I've done a lot of in my life and is an experience I try to avoid at all costs. I had to hide my head behind Richard and look down at my feet on the DuPont escalator because my knees got weak and I started feeling dizzy. (He later climbed up into the Washington monument while I waited down below on trusty solid ground.) If we went today, we'd just budget money for cabs. However, the DuPont Circle area has some good hotels, a big park, nice galleries, lots of little cafés, and some good restaurants. We found that the food in DC was by and large very good, and up to date in terms of interesting ingredients and preparation.

The Lincoln and World War II memorials were inspiring, and I found the names of two of my friends from high school on the Vietnam memorial. Jefferson's memorial has, we thought, the prettiest setting, mimicking his

Virginia home at Monticello. I was thrilled to see the Declaration of Independence and one of four ancient copies of the Magna Carta at the Library of Congress. We particularly liked the National Air and Space Museum, the Museum of Natural History (where I put down my hot pink umbrella on a bench when I rested, got up, walked off without it, and then returned a minute later to recover it and found that it was gone; we kept watching for someone with a vibrant pink umbrella, but the thief had it well hidden . . . so watch your stuff), and the Smithsonian, with its centuries of Americana memorabilia, almost like the biggest garage sale you ever perused. All of those places are on or near The National Mall (the large and long rectangular park in DC—not a shopping mall, though you might think shopping is the American pastime most deserving of a monument). We had lunch in the Smithsonian café, having heard it was a treat, but the food and service were not that good; only the room itself was interesting. We should have known when we walked in that it was not a hot spot, since hardly anyone else was there. This was more than a decade ago, however, so they may have updated the menu (and waitstaff) by now. If not, just go for tea so you can hang out in the room for a half hour or so.

New Orleans

Like DC, New Orleans is a good place—actually, an even better place—to go if you are into music and food. You can hear a lot of music in the French Quarter without walking more than a couple of blocks. Bourbon Street is not as nice as it used to be since the strip joints moved in; Frenchmen's Street (a cab ride away from the Quarter) now has some of the best music clubs and some good restaurants, and we prefer it to Bourbon Street. Of course, there are always music venues accessible by taxi. Some of the van taxis in town accommodate scooters and power chairs. You can also rent a scooter from an equipment rental service, and tool all over the French Quarter. There are a couple of hotels that are not as easy for scooter use, and some are farther away from the Quarter and Jackson Square, so do your research. There's a big Sheraton on the river located conveniently for taking a streetcar along the waterway, down to the Quarter, which can eliminate a long walk.

The Marriott is not a bad place to stay, because there is never a problem getting a taxi from there or back, though it lacks that old French Quarter charm. The Hilton New Orleans Riverside, Four Seasons New Orleans, and Convention Center are right by the Riverfront streetcar line, so you can take a streetcar to the Quarter or the French Market. The St. Charles streetcar can be caught at the west end of Bourbon Street and goes to the Garden District and beyond.

If you can splurge, I recommend the Omni in the Quarter. The least expensive rooms are small, like many rooms in the old section of New Orleans, but everything else about it is great. There's a nice rooftop pool and bar, and a wheelchair lift to the left of the main front door as well. If you park in the basement garage, there's a ramp and elevator to get to the lobby, which we found to be the easiest entrance for a scooter.

A drawback at Le Pavillon Hotel, in addition to its being far from the main part of the French Quarter and needing their personnel to set up ramping at the door if you are using a wheelchair or scooter, is that the pool does not have wheelchair access. But their dinners are excellent, and the rooms are larger than those at some of the other hotels.

There are lots of other places to stay, but, again, do your research. Hotels often change hands or management styles. As for food, don't miss Ralph's in the Garden District for a good dinner. (Some people love their alligator, but I took one bite and thought, *Danger in the swamp!*—too primitive-tasting for me. I passed it over to my husband, who loved it. I thought everything else there was delicious.)

I highly recommend the annual New Orleans Jazz Festival at the county fairground (which is nowhere near the French Quarter), and I'm not a person who generally likes crowds. It's held over two weekends at the end of April and beginning of May. At the festival's main stage, we've seen Joe Cocker, Bruce Springsteen, James Taylor, Irma Thomas, Tom Petty, and the Beach Boys (unfortunately, surf's no longer up, in our opinion), just to name a few. At least one veterans' association offers free push wheelchairs near the entrance, if you have strong arms or someone to push you. (If you use one and can spare the cash, offer a generous contribution in return.) Keep in mind that if you get there after noon, there will probably be no wheelchairs left, because the whole country seems to be on to this free accommodation. There are, yes, thousands of people at the festival, but the fairground is a mammoth, accommodating venue, and we've been twice and absolutely loved it.

There are at least six music venues happening at once at the festival: there's a gospel tent, a jazz stage, a rock-and-roll stage, a zydeco and Cajun music stage, a main stage where the biggest name groups play, and more. Fortunately, the music doesn't conflict; that's how much space there is. The only areas that feel crowded are the fields in front of the main and the rock-and-roll stages, but everyone is generally very relaxed, tolerant, and even friendly—and most of the stages have wheelchair seating near the front, so people in wheelchairs don't end up sitting behind everyone else, unable to see. This is one festival where they have done their best to accommodate disabled people. They even have special, locked, wheelchair-accessible porta-potties; you get a key at the accessibility center not far from the entrance.

In the merchandise area, you'll find vendors selling hats (you'll need one if you have not brought your own), and of course lots of other art tchotchkes and souvenirs. It's not unusual for it to rain in April and May, so slip a poncho into your suitcase, and something to sit on in case you're on one of the many lawns. And, oh yes, there's food. The first time Richard and I went, we discovered the unexpected treat of chicken livers cooked with onions in wine sauce and served with pepper jelly; we also had some crawfish étouffée, and ended our naughty, delicious feast with beignets and café au lait. It wasn't quite on par with the sit-down places in the Quarter or out in the Garden District, but darned good for festival food.

There is a shuttle school bus that goes from a couple of Quarter locations to the fairgrounds. We've found that either taking this shuttle or hiring a bicycle taxi (room for two, and one of the most expensive ways to go, but worth experiencing at least once) is the fastest and most pleasant way to get to and from the festival. Taxis have a hard time getting close to the fairgrounds during the festival and must park a block from the entrances—and from there, it's the equivalent of another block or two into the fairgrounds until you get to the veterans' wheelchairs booth. The buses, in contrast, go onto the fairgrounds themselves and I was able to find a place to sit and wait at the entrance while Richard fetched the wheelchair. When we left, someone from the vets' booth walked to the bus departure area and took the chair back for us. If I went now, of course, I would take my TravelScoot and leave one more wheelchair available for you, if you needed it.

One year at the Jazz Festival, we met a woman I'll call Elise in the small section they have for the many handicapped people who attend the festival. She was probably in her thirties, beautiful, with blond, pixie-cut hair, and was from Utah, where she and her devoted husband had moved because they loved hiking and biking in the great outdoors. She had two kids back home and was frequently texting them when she wasn't swaying to James Taylor.

Elise had lost both her legs above the knee, as well as one arm, in a horrific event. She had no reason to tell me the story in detail—she just said that she'd been in an accident. When we were getting into the van taxi we shared back to our respective hotels after the festival, I put my hands around Elise's waist to pull her into the van as her husband lifted her up and noticed how slim she was.

"Gosh," I said, "how do you stay so tiny? I assume it's pretty hard for you to exercise."

"It has only been a few months since the accident, so this is kind of new to me," she said. "But, small plates. I just order appetizers, never an entree. If I want something from a main course, I have a couple of bites of my husband's."

Good idea, I thought; *maybe I'll try that.* (And I sometimes do).

Encouraged to engage further in conversation, I said, "I had some leg envy at the festival. All those women in shorts and short dresses."

The look she gave me said, *Are you kidding? You've got legs.*

I felt a little twinge of guilt but explained, "It gets tiring, having a paralyzed leg after a few decades. You can't help thinking, *I wish it could have been different, at least for part of my life.*"

No time is a good time to lose function, of course, and we let my comments hang in the air for a pensive moment. But as we neared the Marriott, where they were staying, Elise turned to me again.

"Listen," she said, "you guys have fun tonight. Eat whatever you want. Have a great time. That's what we're doing. You just never know. That's what this experience has taught me—to just do it now, while you can." Then she scooted her pretty self over to the edge of the seat.

"Ready, Elise?" her husband asked.

"Yep!" she said, and he grabbed her waist and lifted her out of the van and onto her scooter.

Laissez les bon temps rouler.

Canada, O Canada

My first trip to Canada was for a conference with The Hunger Project, with whom I was an employee, in the mid-1980s. I fell in love with this cool, green country on that trip, and so was delighted when, fifteen years later, I met online some distant Allen cousins who lived in Toronto and got to go visit them. Canada is a lovely place, in the summer especially, and for us in the United States, such a close and accessible country.

Vancouver, British Columbia, is a charming city, and if you are in the western US, going there is rather like taking an inexpensive trip to a European city where everyone speaks English. (Seattle, Washington, is also a great city to visit, while we're on the subject of beautiful northern towns.) Vancouver has a lot of very nice—and affordable!—hotels and restaurants. Usually, the US dollar is worth 25 percent more in Canada, which means a little luxury will cost less than you'd pay in, say, San Francisco. The last time Richard and I visited Vancouver, we stayed in a two-room suite for a week at Sutton Place Hotel, which was pretty close to perfect and cost about the same as one room at a five-star hotel in San Francisco. Vancouver is also cooler than most of Northern California, so I like to go in the hottest months of the year. If you stay downtown, there's plenty to do, and you can manage to see and enjoy quite a lot with just a small amount of walking.

Stanley Park is a big and beautifully landscaped venue, and I've heard Granville Island, a very short ferry ride away, is also a beautiful place to visit. I found the Museum of Anthropology, with its extensive collection of First Nations artifacts, including totem poles, masks, jewelry and much more, quite remarkable. It's a bit out of the way, so you'll need a rental car or cabs to and from the museum.

Victoria Island is well worth the long ferry ride (and the seemingly interminable wait to get on the ferry with your rental car, both directions; allow for a nearly day-long trip from the mainland to your island destination and the same on your way back). Anyone who loves gardens has absolutely got to see Butchart Gardens, which started about a century ago with a gift to Mrs. Butchart of a packet of sweet pea seeds and a rose bush. This was inspirational to me in that I saw I didn't have to create my garden to be the way I wanted it all at once! Today, Butchart boasts acres of the most remarkable and varied plantings I have ever seen: a rose garden, a Japanese garden, and a Mediterranean garden, just to name a few, and—the most spectacular of all—a park-size garden planted where an old quarry once was operational. You can also go to high tea in the Butcharts' old former residence. I have friends who love the island so much that they fly directly there when they visit, skipping Vancouver and the ferry altogether. Either location is a great vacation; and if you, like me, live in the Pacific time zone, there's no jet lag involved.

The train trip through western Canada, starting from Vancouver and then humming through the Rockies to Lake Louise, is spectacular and worth the pricey fare.

The Rocky Mountaineer is a comfy train with two classes; Richard and I sprang for the more expensive one, since we figured it was a once-in-a-lifetime thing. The scenery was fantastic, the food was fantastic, and a couple of the hotels were, yes, fantastic as well. Generally, we hate tours, because they often involve a lot of walking and a lot of people we think we're not interested in meeting (probably only because we haven't met them!); we do like to socialize, but mostly we travel for scenery, food, music, relaxation, sights, and history. However, on this trip, we found a lot of folks to relate to with widely different backgrounds and persuasions. And since we were riding most of the time, we were rested and had energy to do whatever we wanted to do at each destination.

Whether you live in the northern US and are close enough to drive across the border or live a bit farther south and have to fly, it's a pretty easy proposition to travel to Canada and enjoy a vacay up there. There's a lot to offer—sophisticated cities with great cuisine, breathtaking scenery, and more. If you can't go to Europe and want to fly away, try our neighbor to the north.

⁓

As you can see, the North American continent provides plenty to do and see, some of it even offering a touch of foreign charm. I'd happily return to DC, New Orleans, and parts of Canada more than once in the future to enjoy the food, culture, and sights again. I hope I've inspired you to check them out!

Dear to My Heart—
United Kingdom and Ireland

---oo◯oo---

I've been to England and Scotland, and also Ireland, multiple times. I first went to visit friends in England, then returned and made friends (and met distant relatives) in Scotland and Ireland. I'll never get enough of these bonny islands and their clever people.

Scotland: *Auld Lang Syne*

I grew up believing I was Scottish. The legend was that my dad's family had had a Robert Allen for seven hundred years, my dad being the last (and descended from Robert the Bruce, which many of Scottish ancestry claim, or would like to). When, starting in 1999, I delved deep into my genealogy, I discovered that we have in fact had a Robert Allen in the family since the *1700s*—hence the "seven hundred" reference, handed down incorrectly like a multigenerational game of telephone. I also learned that the Allens were actually in County Wexford, Ireland, not Scotland, from about 1635 to 1925 (though my dad's direct ancestor emigrated to the US in 1793). The family had apparently migrated from England to get away from Cromwell, who promptly followed them to the Emerald Isle—that's what history books say, anyway. We have not yet found roots in England, however, so perhaps they did come from Scotland before either Ireland or England (although they were Protestant, not Catholic, which begs an English connection in the 1550s–1650s).

I learned "The Bonnie Banks o' Loch Lomond" as a small child; my dad whistled it all the time. As to plaid, well, that took a strong position in my closet early on. And bagpipes, of course, those crazily melodic instruments—I love them, can't get enough. Put several together and they make a tear come to this lassie's eye.

Jokes about haggis (and that staple, oat porridge) aside, Scotland also has many good restaurants. Since their economy is partly dependent upon tourism, restaurants and bed-and-breakfast establishments began hiring French chefs or sending their own chefs to French cooking school decades ago, and in a style typical of the Scots, they've adapted the recipes those chefs brought from France to include their traditional fare and local produce, meats, and seafood. You don't have to fear that the cuisine is going to taste like cardboard. And haggis (blood sausage and ground oats, essentially) is actually very tasty, if it's correctly spiced, although I found that I had to eat it sparingly or it had, ahem, a laxative effect.

When Richard invited me to go to Europe with him (mostly a business trip) before our marriage in 1997, Scotland was high on my wish list, and I didn't yet know that I probably wasn't Scottish. So off we went, and I immediately fell in love with Edinburgh and the Scots.

Edinburgh /Auld Reekie (Old Smokey)

Edinburgh ("ED-in-burrah") is ancient, sophisticated, and hip. I guess its nickname is "Auld Reekie" because there used to be a lot of industrial smoke there, but thankfully, that's no longer the case.

There are lots of places in Edinburgh to hear whatever kind of music you crave, including, of course, Scottish traditional, which features fiddle prominently and is one of the bases of bluegrass or hillbilly music (Irish traditional music being the other main base of Anglo-Celtic American roots music, with English folk and madrigal being the third leg to this analogous milking stool). Richard and I particularly like to find a pub with traditional music and slowly sip a wee dram of smooth, slightly smoky, high-quality, single malt whisky. During the annual Edinburgh Festival and the concurrent Edinburgh Fringe Festival in August, it's really easy to find music, theater, or comedy shows to attend, though tickets to the popular classical music and professional theater groups may sell out.

During the festivals, there are also street performers, and you can have a good time walking (or scootering) up and down the High Street, or Royal Mile, and enjoying impromptu shows for no more than a few coins tossed in a performer's basket. Although the streets in Old Town are paved with fairly level brick cobblestones, the sidewalks are flat and smooth and fairly easy to traverse (though some streets involve some fairly steep hills). On our last visit, I found that my TravelScoot served me perfectly there, and the biggest problem I had was that people in crowds tend to stop abruptly or walk directly in front of me when I was accelerating to get up a ramped curb. (Yes, the curbs are ramped at intersections, but the ramping is steep and short, and I needed to get a bit of a running start, leaning forward on my tricycle, to avoid slipping backwards or stalling before I got to level sidewalk. Larger scooters, such as the Pride Go-Go, don't have this issue as much, since they automatically set their brake every time you stop.)

We've stayed at the Radisson Blu on the High Street twice and been totally happy there. It's not often that I have been 100 percent satisfied with a hotel, but this one wins on all fronts. It's as centrally located as an Edinburgh hotel could get, so you don't have to go more than two blocks to find a lot of everything—food, drink, entertainment, and history—and there are no barriers or stairs, as are sometimes found in the older structures in the area. The Balmoral is of course wonderful as well, but it's one of the most expensive hotels not only in Edinburgh but in the world. However, sometimes you can get a substantial discount; we did! Even then it was a splurge, but one we could manage. The staff at either place will take excellent care of you, and both venues have very nice indoor pools. The food's very good; there is more than one restaurant at each of those hotels, with other café and restaurant choices on the streets nearby.

Down the hill and around the corner from the Radisson Blu, on North Bridge Street, there's a little tea shop, Patisserie Valerie, that has a variety of very good pastries. About a block or two up the Royal Mile, there is an elegant tearoom behind St. Giles' Cathedral churchyard; we were never able to coordinate times with them, but I'm told they have a very lovely high tea. Our favorite foodie restaurant in that area is Angels with Bagpipes, across the street from St. Giles'. There are no bagpipes playing, but there's a large angel statue inside, and all their entrees and wines are excellent. If you want to try an updated, tasty haggis, they have a great appetizer (the haggis appetizer at the Radisson Blu is a close second).

The annual Military Tattoo (nothing to do with inked skin, although you're likely to see a lot of that in Edinburgh) is also held nightly during the festival at the Edinburgh Castle Esplanade, with hundreds of bagpipes involved. A number of countries are represented there in colorful traditional or updated costumes, performing as marching bands, other musical groups, and dancers. There's a very professional and artistic light show projected onto the castle at the same time, so, lots of treats for the senses. Several thousand people go each evening; it's wise to get tickets at least a month or two in advance.

There is a special rate and special seating for those in wheelchairs or on scooters at the Military Tattoo; the handicapped person may pay full price but a companion— or "carer," as they call them in the UK—gets in free. Sometimes tickets are still available two or three weeks prior to the night you wish to go. However, a caution: if your Disabled Person tickets are not mailed to you three weeks or more before the event, you have to pick them up—in person—at the Tattoo office in Edinburgh, which is at the bottom of a very, very steep hill, many blocks from the venue itself, and difficult to access (almost impossible for a wheelchair)!

Taxis or self-driven autos with special permits you obtain with your tickets are the only ones allowed up at the castle on the nights of the Tattoo, but your cab will wait a long time in line, which cranks up the taxi fee, and a personal driver will almost certainly need to leave and come back later, since so little parking is available. When Richard and I went, we paid the high fee to take a cab up the long, steep hill, partly because it was drizzling and we would have had to wait outside for an hour. Afterward, we skipped getting a ride, given the rain had stopped, and joined the throngs of spectators leaving the castle gates—me scootering and Richard walking—to head the mile back down the hill to our hotel.

There are quite a few Edinburgh galleries and museums you may wish to visit; I've been to the two-building complex of the Scottish National Gallery of Modern Art and the Scottish National Gallery, as well as Edinburgh Castle, which all have exceptionally good gift shops with Scottish or UK art, crafts, and wares. Getting to the castle is quite an endeavor; you can take a cab up to it (there are a very few DP parking spaces up there), and then the hiking around in the castle is pretty extensive. A few wheelchairs are available, but they are hard to push on the cobbled streets and walkways within the castle. A mobility vehicle may be available if you book it in advance, and you can also bring your own scooter. It's worth a try if you have any interest in Scottish ancient history, as it's the best restored castle I've seen—and I've seen a couple of dozen at least.

Another castle that is far more accessible is Holyrood, the Queen of England's residence when she stays in Edinburgh, at the lower end of the Royal Mile/High Street. There are push wheelchairs available, and elevators, and a tearoom. The gift shop is a very good place to buy cards with excellent old prints, I found. If the queen (or king) is in residence, of course, you won't be able to visit the castle itself.

Glasgow/Dear Green Place

Glasgow has the Glasgow School of Art, founded by Charles Rennie Mackintosh, who was also its Art Nouveau architect. Tours have been available at specified times, and the gift and card shop are very good; I got some Art Nouveau number stencils there that we used to fashion our house numbers at home. However, the main part of the school suffered an extensive fire in 2018, so I would check to see if renovations have been made before deciding to visit (they may not be complete until 2028). On the plus side, there was no ramp to the entrance of the school before, only stairs, and there is intention to make the building more accessible during the renovation.

The Mackintosh House in the Hunterian Museum at University of Glasgow is a real treat for those who revere the artist and designer. (This also involved stairs; I am a huge fan of Mackintosh, however, so I was determined.) You can google his name and see a little of his artwork; you may have that "aha!" moment wherein you realize you're familiar with his designs but didn't know they were his, and also feel, as I did, that you just have to see the Mackintosh House. His interior designs have been partially recreated there.

We took the train to Glasgow from Edinburgh on an intermittently rainy day (common in Scotland), and found that there were few taxis available at the Glasgow train station (not the main one but the one in the neighborhoods of the school and university), nor at the School of Art, or the University. So we did a lot of walking, which was difficult then; I would not be able to do that today. It might be more realistic with a scooter, but I'd recommend renting a car and driving from Edinburgh, if that's your starting point, unless walking is not an issue for you. I understand that Glasgow also has a lot of traditional and current music venues, so it might even be worth an overnight stay. It has a reputation as a rather rough town—Denise Mina, the Scottish mystery writer, says with tongue in cheek that everyone in Glasgow knows someone who's been in jail—but it is also full of artists and musicians.

Out to the (Amazing) Country

The areas north and far west of Edinburgh should not be missed if you have more than a couple of days in Scotland. The first time we were in Edinburgh, we were overwhelmed by the throngs gathered there for the arts festival, partly because we were not prepared for the scarcity of taxis and I didn't have a scooter. When the concierge at the hotel, picking up on our fatigue, asked us if we had been out of town, we answered that we hadn't, and he said, "If this is your first trip to Scotland and you only have a few days, you really should take a car and go out into the highlands. It would be a shame not to see the country." And that's just what we did; we drove for a couple of days and spontaneously stayed at one bed-and-breakfast in the lochs region.

There's a vista point on the way from Glasgow to Loch Lomond with a sign that reads, REST AND BE THANKFUL. The view of the glen is so peaceful and awe-inspiring, you can't help but do as the name suggests.

This was a lot of driving in a short time, so on our next trips we took trains and rented cars when we arrived at our destinations.

The three-hour train trip from Edinburgh to Inverness and back is a lovely one, and it's far more restful than the long drive. One year we had an amusing time standing in line waiting for our car at the train station in Inverness. The day was typically misty, and the fellow in front of us complained to the lass at the rental car counter about what a disappointment it was to him. She wryly replied, "Well, ye don't come to Scotland for the weather now, do ye?"

No, you don't, I could have told the man. You come for the spectacular scenery, the light in the summer, the music—especially the *ceilidhs* ("KAY-leehs"), music parties at pubs or homes—the art, the gardens, the history, the food, the Scotch, the peace, the well-paved roads with sane drivers, and the camaraderie. I think that'd be sufficient to make up for a bit o' mist.

The highland scenery is some of the most awesome on the planet. Huge cliffs dropping to clear rivers or the sea itself, mountains covered in green and creased with an occasional rocky waterfall, with glens or valleys cradling myriad lakes (lochs) and rivers. I am particularly fond of the Summer Isles area near Ullapool (northwest), the lochs area near Loch Lomond and Kilmartin, and Inverness (which has some excellent restaurants, including Rocpool and White House, and a couple of good music venues, Hootenanny being our favorite).

The Isle of Skye is another beautiful place, though sparse in accommodation, that's accessed by ferry from Kyle of Lochalsh. When we were on Skye, we went to a bagpiping competition which turned out to be only of the peabroch style, which is lamenting, and for our American ears, was a bit difficult to listen to for hours. There was, fortunately, in the middle of it, a recital by some girls from a music school in Loch Lomond, and they were fantastic. If we were ever going to the Loch Lomond area again, we'd check out whether that school would have any concerts or recitals. We also like Perth, where we stayed at one of the loveliest B and B's in the UK, and the Kingdom (county) of Fife, just north of Edinburgh, where the little town of Achtermuchty puts on a decent music and art festival annually. Aberdeen has a very good annual music fest as well, perhaps even better.

One of Scotland's most spectacular resources, however, is its people. Nearly everyone we've met there has been friendly, helpful, of good humor, and smart. We were particularly moved when some friends there said, upon our departure, "Haste ye back." This comes from a Scottish verse that goes, approximately, "Haste ye back, we loue [love] you dearly . . ."

I'm ready to hasten back the minute I leave.

Ireland: *Slainte!*

The Irish say, "*Slainte!*" ("SLAHN-juh")—"To your health!"—before tipping a pint.

I visited Ireland with Richard for the first time before I knew that my dad's family was actually Irish. I loved Dublin; we stayed at the Westbury, which is just behind Grafton Street, a primary shopping walk. It's a nice venue, and the only reason we didn't stay there again was that it doesn't have a pool, and a few other hotels in Dublin do. (If I don't get in a pool once or twice a week, I typically have considerable back trouble.)

One of the hotels *with* pool that we've discovered is the Shelbourne, right on St. Stephen's Green. The convoluted path up and down the stairs and hallways to the pool is extremely inconvenient, but they serve a great high tea. The Merrion, meanwhile, is expensive and a bit over-rated—and it requires a person with walking difficulty to have a scooter or wheelchair to get to the far reaches of the hotel rooms themselves—but the pool is really great. Their high tea is way over the top in terms of sugar content; I've never seen so many sweets in one meal, and we took a small box away with us. The Westin is one of our favorites but, like the Westbury, has no pool, so in my case it's good only for one or two nights—usually when we fly in and out of Dublin. (There are also far less expensive hotels in the area that I'm sure are perfectly comfortable; we have never stayed more than a couple of nights in Dublin, so each time we've gone, we've decided on luxury.)

The Temple Bar Pub in the Temple Bar neighborhood is the most famous, most crowded, and most likely to have good traditional music of any pub in Dublin, though some of their music is not as traditional as one might hope. Just be prepared to stand up in one of the warren rooms until someone staggers out or some kind person gives up their stool or chair—a favor that's somewhat likely if you come in on crutches or with a cane. O'Donoghue's, which is right near the Merrion, also has nightly traditional music; we found it to be no less crowded than the Temple Bar Pub, but it seemed people came and went more often, so nabbing a spot near the musicians' session corner was a little more likely. On two visits, we also found the musicians there to be better than the ones we heard at The Temple Bar Pub, so there you go. The Temple Bar area is not easy walking—lots of cobblestones and narrow sidewalks. I was able to make do with my TravelScoot, but Richard had to help me lift it up and down curbs a few times—so if you cannot get out of a wheelchair, there will be limited streets and venues in that neighborhood that you can access.

Since my dad's ancestral family had a large farm in County Wexford for two hundred years, we've been down there a few times. We struck up an ongoing friendship with the current owner and also a former church docent, who helped me log my family's copious genealogical data from the local parish records. Wexford Town has a big harbor, some interesting history, and some good restaurants (The Yard is our favorite), and like Dublin, the going is a little rough there, but my motorized trike was manageable with a little help. The hotels there are not top-notch (Clayton White's was a particular blight on our last trip) but Talbot's is pretty good, and locals have told me that Whitford House and Ferrycarrig Hotel are much better than Clayton White's, but they're two miles from the town center. If you can do stairs, there are some good bed-and-breakfasts.

We attended an arts festival in Kilkenny, located in the south-central area of Ireland. It's a pretty drive from whatever point you start, and the town itself is billed as "the most medieval city in Ireland." The castle and cathedral there are formidable and elegant, particularly the cathedral, where we heard the festival's closing concert, which featured classical, jazz, traditional Irish, bluegrass, country and also some poetry accompanied by music. The festival is in August each year and includes plays and comedy as well, all of it impressive. The town itself is charming, too, and I scootered around fairly easily to the cafés and other venues there. We stayed at Kilkenny River Court hotel on John Street, which was quite pleasant and convenient. I'd definitely go back there, especially during the festival.

We also enjoyed Cork, and the little town of Kinsale— south of there, on the coast—was as pretty as they come, with a well-earned reputation for having the best foodie food in Ireland. We found that even the pub food in

Kinsale was excellent—and sometimes even accompanied by traditional music and singalongs.

I do hope I get to Ireland again; I haven't yet seen the western coast or Northern Ireland!

England: *Cheerio*

In England, we primarily go to visit friends who used to live in the west, and on our visits, we've enjoyed a number of lovely western sights. Glastonbury—both its town, with the ancient peaceful Lady Well and its bookshops, and especially the old abbey, where, legend has it, King Arthur is buried—is an exceptional place. Stonehenge, with its mysterious impressive standing stones, Lacock Abbey, used in the Harry Potter films, Highclere Castle, where the Downton Abbey series was filmed (and which has a fabulous garden downhill from the castle), Oxford University, and Bath ("Bahth"), with its Roman baths and art galleries, are all places not to miss if you find yourself one to three hours west of London. There are a number of excellent Indian restaurants in Oxford, we were pleased to learn (and enjoy). I thought when I saw the film *The Man Who Knew Infinity* that the famed genius Indian mathematician Srinivasa Ramanujan was one-and-a-half centuries too early at Cambridge, because he could not find vegetarian food in the UK in the early 1900s.

Brighton, south of London, with its seaside walks and flamboyant castle, and Cambridge, with its university and its church where you can make a rubbing of old carved motifs (the one I did is of a raucous Green Man and his woody environment, metallic gold crayon on black paper, and now hangs in our front hall), are both worth a day's visit as well.

Restaurants, shopping, and shows in London ("Theatreland," in and near the West End, is the district for shows) can be really fun; plus there are galleries, museums, and the Royal Ballet. (I saw *Swan Lake* one afternoon at the Royal Opera House—really a treat.) The downtown area is fairly flat but is not my favorite place in which to spend time, although now that I have a scooter I might find it more pleasant. Personally, I'd rather spend my time out in the country or in one of the pretty neighboring towns than in the big city. But if you're a theater and shopping buff, you will likely love London.

Again, take note of where you're going to be in the British Isles before you fly in, because Heathrow is a huge airport and takes a lot of time to navigate. Airports at Stansted, Birmingham, Norwich, Exeter, or Edinburgh may serve you as well or better. However, some of the smaller airports have baggage limitations because they accommodate smaller planes, so if you are bringing a scooter, check on all of that before booking.

Doing my best royal wave here, as we depart the British Isles. Ta-ta, and cheerio!

Farther Afield—
India, Egypt, and Israel

━━━━━━━━━━○○○○○━━━━━━━━━━

1 traveled to these places with a group of Sufis in the early 1980s. Though we were on a tight budget, we were able to have a great time. Our purpose was to meet with other Sufi teachers and do singing practices together, but we fully enjoyed being tourists "on the cheap." If I returned to any of these one day, it would probably be to India, and I'd stay in one or more of the many nicer hotels they offer.

India

India is not a bad choice as a foreign travel destination for western handicapped people with a little money. The hotels are inexpensive compared to those in western countries, and the cities, though crowded, have *tuk tuks*—those covered, three-wheeled scooter taxis. Speedy, careening, and occasionally frightening as they might be, they'll take you everywhere you want to go cheaply. Even so, be prepared for everything to take longer than you're used to; in my experience traveling there, there's no use being in a hurry.

There is notable stigma about disability in India. Many of the Indian people who are handicapped and out on the streets are referred to as "untouchables"—people from the lowest castes living in abject poverty. When I visited the country, I didn't see handicapped people out and about very much, because in 1982, there was not the funding for assistive devices that we have always had here. In China, too, it was not until the 1960s that there was any funding for disabled people. Handicapped citizens were not educated, because it was thought that they would never be useful, even if they were intelligent. Even parents of blind children did not teach them basic skills, thinking that they had no future other than to beg. Thanks to the work in China of people like Mu Mengjie, who was blind from birth and started a school for blind children, attention has been brought to the potential that handicapped children and adults can meet if given the tools. Although both India and China are still challenged as to resources, accommodation, and inclusion for disabled people, both countries are making an attempt to right this.

I realize now that people stared at me in India in the early 1980s not only because I was Western and strange to them, but also because I was handicapped and able to travel at all. Marriage is a sacred institution there; a husband has to be able to work to support his family and a wife must be able to do the domestic chores, and perhaps also work outside the home. So, it was not unusual that I should be single—the assumption would have been that this was because I was lame—but for me to be able to travel at all put me in the category of "rich woman." (Not actually the case, of course, at least not by US standards: I had borrowed the money to take this three-month trip, five weeks of it in India, and it took me two or three years to pay it back. Still, a woman with polio in India at that time would have been dependent upon her family or working as a servant, and probably would not even have had the resources to borrow money to travel, so my seemingly lucky circumstance was a curiosity to the Indian people I encountered.)

Many polio patients in India are reduced to begging and/or being untouchables, unless they become nuns or live in some type of spiritual community. However, the current government is making a concerted effort to supply handicapped people with bracing so that children do not become more crippled and adults are able to function and work. I met one lovely woman there, a polio survivor, who worked as a devoted assistant to a saintly Vedantic teacher in southern India. Unfortunately, since she didn't speak English, and the only word I know in Hindi is "ek" (one), I did not get to swap stories with her.

I have met two Indian polio survivors here in the US. Both of them contracted polio from the vaccine administered in India in the last half of the twentieth century, which was oral and live. At that time, it was difficult and expensive to provide inoculation equipment, assure the necessary refrigeration, and train medical personnel how to administer the shots, (plus pay them), especially in remote, widespread, and hot rural areas (as has been true in African countries also). Inoculations only use dead vaccine, which is safer. With live vaccine, there is an extremely low risk of people coming down with the disease because it contains live virus—but while polio was at epidemic proportions, the risk of getting the disease itself was considered a far higher and far worse one.

Unfortunately, people like the ones I met here in the US were collateral damage of that oral vaccination program—and since they also did not have access to the great bracing, rehab, and physical therapy I've been privileged to take advantage of, they now deal with worse, lingering effects.

Today, everywhere in the world, the move toward killed, inoculated vaccine has been initiated, and India has not had a new case of polio in nearly a decade.

Exploring India

I had a great time in New Delhi, Jaipur, and Agra, home of the Taj Mahal (another sight I think that everyone should see), traveling with Sufi friends on our long spiritual trek. It was nice to take things slower, see shrines and art, hear music, and go to restaurants that we, in those days, would not have been able to afford in the West. One of these was the Imperial Hotel, where we ate like kings on one occasion and even ordered baked Alaska, which I had never had in my youth and which seemed exotic to me at the time. We were even able to pay a small sum to come and use the outdoor pool there, which had waiters accommodating us with drinks service—the height of luxury for a bunch of ex-hippies in our thirties. The restaurant at the Imperial has been updated since our visit, but is now pretty far down on the list of great places to eat in New Delhi. Still, the old hotel itself is grand and worth a visit, whether you eat there or not.

We also ate at Gaylord Restaurant, an international chain with traditional Indian fare, more than once during our time in New Delhi. The most interesting aspect to us was that they employed so many people. One person greeted us at the door, another showed us to our seats, another took our orders, someone else delivered drinks, someone else delivered the food, another worker was using a carpet sweeper while we ate, and so on. It was a nice alternative to our US multitasking, hire-as-few-people-as-possible standards—though the practice does feed into the hierarchy of the caste system. One of the places we stayed in Delhi was the YMCA hostel. That was a very inexpensive place where we used a communal bathroom, with men having certain hours and women the other times, and which was kept sanitized with an overpowering, nose-assaulting kerosene disinfectant. We slept three beds to a room, which worked well in terms of keeping our costs down. There was a modest restaurant which served three meals daily and SNACKS, as the café sign announced, in the late afternoon. Today, the YMCA tourist hotel is much, much nicer; the pictures of the lobby have updated furniture and lighting.

I found that for most of the time in India, I felt a little poorly, with indigestion or worse, and that what settled my stomach was beer (which I had not liked before, but I learned to like Kingfisher and Taj Mahal) and potato chips! Given that I generally eat a wholesome diet, this was a surprise turn for me, but I think the salt helped me to feel less light-headed in the heat, and the beer for some reason was the right thing for my tummy. I may have accidentally ingested some water with a bug in it, even though we made our best effort never to drink unboiled or untreated water, having brought small portable water filtration systems. (FYI, the more upscale the restaurant, the more likely the water, including the ice, will be filtered.) All that to say, I now enjoy a beer occasionally! We also drank a lot of lime sodas, made with fresh lime juice, soda water, and sugar, fruit lassis (LAH-see)—a delicious drink made of yogurt, ice, and fruit—and cold coffee ice creams, which were essentially coffee floats with chocolate or vanilla ice cream. Yum!

In Delhi, since this was not so much a vacation as a spiritual trek, we primarily visited Sufi shrines and sang there, which was entertaining for the Indian Sufis in that our Arabic chants were jazzier than their traditional ones. They also were surprised to find that in our group, the women sang as well, and often carried the melodies. Unfortunately, this attitude has not changed much in recent decades; women are often considered "less than" by many male Indians, and indeed, it's not always a good idea for a woman to be on the streets alone unless it's the middle of the day and you're in well-populated areas such as shopping districts, hotels, or nicer restaurants. I took scooter taxis alone a few times while I was there, but I didn't think it was a good idea to take a bus alone.

There are large numbers of orphan children in India, and many of them are disabled. It's a disturbing thing to see if one is not prepared for it, but solutions are being pursued and it's possible to contribute to charities that assist orphans to transition to a normal life by providing them with real stability, rather than the squalor that can exist in some orphanages in India. (Some of these non-profits are US-based; please see my Resources section for three that I recommend.) Contributing in this way may help alleviate any concern that might keep you from enjoying India's vibrant cultures.

In Jaipur, the big draw was the Amber Fort, where we rode elephants up the very steep road to the top and visited the Kali shrine, and I bought a small emerald down in one of the jewelry area shops since the town is known for its reasonably priced gemstones. I would not have been able to see the famous fort if I'd had to walk up the very steep hill, so the ride was essential. There is an ongoing movement to stop the elephant rides, which are considered cruel treatment of the gentle creatures—something my friends and I did not know at the time of our trip. Today, you can also reach the top by Jeep, golf cart, or your own vehicle (none of which were options for us when we were there).

Agra of course has the Taj Mahal, a shrine to the beloved wife of the Shah Jehan, Mumtaz Mahal. We sang our chants there one evening, enthralled by how the music reverberated in the marble hall, and I took advantage of the emptiness of the Taj in the early morning one day and sang there alone. Pictures of the Taj do not do it justice.

The mosaic work and the symmetry of the dome are best appreciated in person, and it's one of those sights that is well worth the long flight to India.

Egypt

My travel in Egypt took place long before the populist uprisings in the early 2000s and their accompanying riots, governmental changes, and political turmoil, which is still at issue today—so I'm glad I went when I did. If you have a deeply adventurous spirit, you may want to go anyway, but be sure to check to see if Egypt is on a list of places our State Department recommends we avoid before you get excited and book a trip.

Egypt in the 1980s was an interesting place to visit. Cairo, Alexandria, and Saqqaro were particularly fascinating. The Egyptian museum in Cairo requires three days of exploration and is conveniently located near a good western hotel that occasionally changes ownership; it was a Hilton when I was there. Tutankhamen's remains are there (in the museum, not the hotel); they're pretty awe-inspiring, and what a case they built for him. It's as magnificent as it looks in any pictures you've seen. And there are lots (and lots) of other mummies and spectacular artifacts on every floor.

Cairo's Coptic churches are among the most ancient Christian structures in the world and contain some exceptional early art, and of course there are the pyramids at Giza, and the Sphinx, just outside of Cairo. It's possible to go into one of the pyramids and enter a tunnel deep into its center; however, the friends I was traveling with said that one must walk bent over all the way in, so I skipped this experience. Some relatives of mine who went recently said they had the same bent-over walk and it was pretty difficult, especially for people in their seventies. If you are able to walk while bent at the waist, are not claustrophobic, and are curious, you might try it, but I don't think it's a venue designed for the handicapped traveler. Horses are available to ride a little way into the desert sands between the three pyramids, accompanied by local guides, if you are an equestrian.

Boat cruises on the Nile and carriage rides in Cairo provide relaxing, physically undemanding diversions. Mohamed Ali mosque is beautiful and immense and worth a reverent look inside; be sure to wear a head covering and remove your shoes, and if you speak at all, do so in a whisper. People go there to pray five times a day and sometimes in between.

Unfortunately, Cairo also has the worst pollution, partly due to coal fires and diesel vehicles, that I have ever experienced, even compared to Los Angeles (when it had its worst heavy smog). But the museum is worth tolerating the air or lack thereof. Stay away from the bazaar, where a British friend's passport was stolen from her tote bag while she strolled along shopping. (It was frustratingly complicated for her to get another one there in Cairo, too, even with the help of the British embassy.) My experience with the cab drivers in Cairo was that they were seemingly without scruples, usually doubling or tripling fees for us Westerners. Luckily, some Egyptians waiting for cabs with us told us, in English, "They are exploiting you; ride with us," and would not take reimbursement when we disembarked. The Egyptians we met, other than those cab drivers and the military folks at the airports, were very kind and helpful.

Alexandria, on the Mediterranean Sea, a pleasant three-hour train ride from Cairo, is beautiful, clean, and has a surprisingly excellent though small tropical aquarium, some good cafés, and Roman ruins well worth seeing. Saqqaro is about an hour's drive outside of Cairo. It boasts columns and crypts that are more detailed (with lots of intact hieroglyphs) and in better condition than the three pyramids at Giza. I stood on the tomb of a princess in the crypts at Saqqaro. When the stone started to vibrate with no discernible cause, and no one else felt the buzzing, I jumped off, a bit alarmed. I didn't draw any conclusions (although it was easy to think the ancient princess didn't want me standing on her crypt), but the experience did impress me.

As I'm writing this in late 2020, much of the Arab world in Africa is not safe for travel. I hope that one day things will be settled and peaceful there. I believe we have more in common than we have differences; most everyone loves his or her family and friends and wishes for a tranquil, happy life. I try to remember this when looking beyond my own life to other cultures.

Israel

Israel is clean and a great place to tour, though it is hilly and rocky, and some areas have a lot of stairs. Something I appreciated was that the buses in Jerusalem were reliable—and on top of that there were always at least eight people at every bus stop, and one of them always spoke English and was happy to tell me if I was getting on the right bus.

The old city of Jerusalem is a treasure. If you need to visit a particular shop, keep in mind that you will need to know the religion of the shopkeeper. Muslim vendors close Thursday night and all-day Friday; Jewish vendors close Friday night and all-day Saturday; and Christian vendors are closed on Sunday. I was in awe of the variety of merchandise available there, but even more so with the excavations being done, which have revealed centuries of cities built upon cities.

When my friends and I visited Israel in the 1980s, we also saw the spot on the Mount where Christ was supposed to have ascended, complete with a vague, rocky footprint, and visited the Garden of Gethsemane, where nearby a Hassidic or Orthodox fellow did his davening prayers near the gravesite of a loved one. Another religious site is said to be the tomb of Rabia, who was a Muslim holy woman. After finding a caretaker who had a key to the tomb, we women enjoyed a peaceful meditation inside surrounded by forest green drapery—the color associated with Islam, which symbolizes Paradise.

It's relatively easy for a handicapped person to get around in Jerusalem, Tel Aviv (nice beach, nice hotels), and other parts of Israel—as long as you avoid the rocky hillsides. So if you've a desire to go, it's an accessible, and beautiful, place to tour. Shalom!

Scary Stories!

Travel's not always easy. Following are some experiences I've had that are a bit absurd; perhaps they'll either make you laugh or make your jaw drop. (Spoiler alert: this includes alarming experiences you may never have and can probably avoid.)

Terminal Nightmares

As I mentioned in Chapter 2, foreign airports, and other venues as well, tend to have less accommodation for passengers in wheelchairs than we have in the US. This may be because we have the Americans with Disabilities Act, which requires that handicapped people be able to get to the same places as normies.

At Heathrow in London, I had one connecting flight that was in a different terminal, probably a mile or more from the gate where we disembarked from our arriving flight. I had been told it was a "short walk" when I got off the plane, but it wasn't; it was far beyond my ability. I suppose a mile is a short walk for a European, or a normal person; but as I've probably made clear by now, if *I* walk a mile, I will need to stop and rest at least ten times and probably sit down for a few minutes along the way. Don't assume people will notice your manual wheelchair, crutches, or cane, and put it together that any walk is a long walk for you. In that instance I had to flag down one of those electric carts the airlines use for staff in the corridor, or I would have missed my plane—and before that a few carts passed me and did not ask if I wanted a lift, even though I was using a cane and was visibly under stress.

Another time, upon arriving at Heathrow my husband and I had to go up and down several flights of stairs, even though I had said I needed a wheelchair and we had an attendant accompanying us. We got to a point in the walk where they asked me to get up out of the chair and walk the rest of the way, which included stairs. I looked at the attendant incredulously; I can climb stairs, fortunately, with great difficulty, but some people can't do this at all. I don't know what her plan was for those in our entourage who couldn't walk, because this was where we parted company. This incident may have been due to the short-sightedness of the attendant, who did not think to take me on a route where there was an elevator. But generally, all the attendants take you on the same route. They want and need to make their job as easy for themselves as possible.

Today, Heathrow attendants appear to understand that any route with stairs is unrealistic for disabled travelers. Perhaps they've hired more astute attendants, or they've started giving them a course on our needs and abilities before sending them out into the terminals, but I have not had anyone even suggest that we take stairs in our last few trips through Heathrow.

Once, at Charles de Gaulle airport outside Paris, I was dumped from a wheelchair on a ramped moving sidewalk onto the floor by an inexperienced attendant. I wasn't hurt, but clearly, he had not practiced and was not up to the task. It was like something out of a comedic movie; all of a sudden, I was on the floor on my hands and knees, right at the end of the ramp, with others approaching at moving-ramp speed behind us. Again, fortunately, I can get up from a floor since I do floor yoga every morning. But it's not easy, especially after the shock of a fall. I was imagining a pileup of people, but they were far enough behind us that with Richard's help, I, the attendant, and the wheelchair were able to move quickly out of the way. But what a fiasco.

Another time, at Charles de Gaulle in 2008, we and several other handicapped people and their companions were asked to wait until all other passengers had disembarked, and then were herded from the back exit door of the plane into a hot and stuffy elevated cage on the back of a truck and kept there for a half-hour. Next, we were ferried all over the airport for an hour, dropping a couple of our caged companions for their connecting flights. When the rest of us were finally deposited in an empty terminal ourselves, there were no wheelchairs (or passengers, except us, for that matter) left at that location. There were supposed to be attendants to take us to baggage claim; instead, there was one airport employee who didn't know when the terminal would be in use again—"When there's another flight from here," he blandly told us. So, we were expected to wait, and wait, and wait.

Finally, after at least a half hour (on top of the previous sixty to ninety minutes we'd lost touring the airport in a cage!), we six handicapped people and some spouses revolted and walked about two miles through various terminals to the baggage claim, frequently stopping to rest, defying the multiple checkpoint security guards who said it was out of order for us to do so. They didn't have guns, so they were helpless when confronted by our united crippled will to get out of the airport. I think the French among us were a little titillated by this rebelling against authority. (The French are generally very orderly and accepting of rules, in my limited observance.) It took us an hour to walk the mile or so to the baggage claim area, where our bags were circulating over and over out to the loading dock and back in on the conveyor belt, but we were relieved we'd made it and that the bags were all still there.

One Frenchman had badly broken his foot the day before in New York City. He was on crutches and on his way home to Paris. An ambulance was waiting outside the baggage area to take him to a hospital. The airport personnel understood this. The traveler did not complain; he knew there was no use complaining about French systems. So I limped along, pushing his luggage cart with my walking sticks balanced on top, while he gingerly maneuvered on his new crutches and Richard pushed our cart. Fortunately, the ambulance driver did wait the two hours for this poor fellow, which surprised me. Probably the ambulance was dispatched and paid for by the government; in the US, where ambulances are privately owned, he would have had to call a second one.

When we returned home, I wrote letters to Charles De Gaulle airport, the airline, and the handicapped people's organization in Paris and complained about this debacle. Months passed, and eventually I got a letter from the airport saying, "Not our fault, so sorry, the airlines handle all their own disabled-person transport in the airport. *But we're changing all that next year, and the airport will in the future be handling all the transport in all terminals, so things should be better coordinated." Well, nice*, I thought. *Assuming we ever wanted to fly into that airport again.* But then, much later, another letter arrived from the airline (a result of my having written to the airport and the Parisian disabled person's organization, I suspected), accompanied by two vouchers good for about $300 apiece for our next trip with them, with an expiration date about a year out. Squeaky wheel got some good grease. And we did use them, happy to say.

On that subsequent trip to France in 2009, we made plans to meet friends at the train station closest to CDG airport when we arrived from the US for a trip to the south of France. This time, we were again asked to wait until every single blankety-blank passenger was off the plane, but this time I refused, since I did not need a transfer chair. To the airport's credit, the letter I'd received from CDG a year or two before was true: their policies had changed. A wheelchair and attendant arrived at the gate within a very short time, and the lovely young woman said, "Oh, yes, yes; it's not far"; she could take us to the train station adjacent to the airport.

The attendant helped us collect our luggage and took us to the far end of the airport near the train station—near, but not near enough, about a quarter- to a half-mile away—and said, "Sorry, I cannot take you further." So we walked the long remaining distance, unable to take the cart any further—Richard grappling with the luggage while I pushed one piece and used my crutch on the other side. Had we known she could not take us the full distance, we'd have had her take us to baggage claim, then gone outside the airport, and taken a taxi to the train station. But at least we know now.

Quel Dommage (What a Pity)

We were on a flight to France. Dinner had just been delivered to all of us, and I was ready to tuck in to what looked like a nice meal, when the woman in front of me decided to raise her head rest . . . . which kept right on rising, came flying off the top of the supports, did a back flip, and landed on my tray. Food was all over the place—on me, my purse, my carry-on bag, the floor, the window. I exclaimed something probably not fit for publication and put my sauce-soaked hands up, since there was nothing I could touch without making more of a mess.

The headrest sat there on top of my dinner, acting innocent. The woman in the faulty seat stood up, turned around, looked at me, and smiled; Richard handed her the errant headrest; and she sat back down again. No "sorry" or "*desolé*" escaped her lips. She called an attendant and two of them scurried about, trying to figure out what to do; I think they told her she'd just have to go without a headrest, since it was clearly broken.

But what about me, covered in dinner? Richard called for an attendant.

A tall blond woman responded and saw the mess; we told her about the mishap. "Oh, sorry," she said, "would you like a glass of champagne?"

"Yes, *oui*," I replied, "but first I'd like a rag or some napkins to clean up this mess." She disappeared and never returned (and, insult to injury, the promise of champagne was not kept). When we realized she wasn't coming back, Richard grabbed a handful of napkins from the galley so I could at least wipe my hands. Then he waved to another attendant.

This one was short, blond, pretty, and friendly to the French people with whom she was carrying on a patter of chatter. We showed her the mess, told her it was a result of the broken headrest of the passenger in front of me and that I had not gotten my meal, and said we would like to clean it all up as soon as possible.

All friendliness gone, the attendant said, "Yes, Madame, you just sit here quietly until the flight is over and we will clean it up then," and walked away.

There were seven hours left to go in the flight.

Richard went to the galley again and got a rag and we cleaned up the mess, and then, gallant gentleman that he is, he shared his dinner with me.

I was quietly appalled and furious. What a start to a much-anticipated trip to Paris.

As we disembarked the plane eight sleepy hours later, I quickly discovered that I had left my prescription reading glasses in the little glasses clip on the back of the seat with the flying headrest. As soon as we knew this, we advised the Air France people at the gate and they said they'd look on the plane (once we determined what to call "glasses," because at first no one knew what we were talking about, even though they all spoke English). They came back to us and said, "No, no spectacles, sorry." The clean-up crew was still on the plane; I couldn't believe they would not have seen the glasses hanging on the back of a seat, especially with our specific seat numbers in hand. I asked if they had a lost and found, and they gave me a phone number, which we called daily from our hotel until I finally gave up. Eyeglasses are sellable on the black market, and although these were prescription, I'm sure someone is happily wearing my pink wire-framed readers.

Moral of the story: No matter how sleepy you are, don't leave the plane until you scan every square inch of your seating area for your belongings—seatback pocket and under both your seat and the one in front of you, especially. That airline is one of the few that has eyeglass clips, so it was easy to forget that I'd utilized the unusual convenience when I gathered up my stuff.

Meanwhile, back in the Far East . . .

It's been thirty-seven years since I traveled with Indian Air, but those two flights were the most terrifying I've ever had. When we landed at Bangalore, there was a cliff at the end of the short runway, and we were gripping our armrests in anticipation of a potential crash over the precipice. On our way back to Delhi, a couple of us were not wearing our seatbelts during part of the trip. At one point we encountered some extreme turbulence quite suddenly, with no warning from the captain. Before I had time to even think of buckling up, I was ejected out of my seat and my head hit the ceiling of the aircraft while at the same time, I kid you not, my tea jumped out of my cup and back into it! (Well, some of it ended up on the tray table, of course.) I've never had an experience approaching these, before or since, on any airline.

Ou Est Ma Valise?! (Where's My Suitcase?!)

On that same French messy-meal-lost-glasses-flight vacation, we'd made a pretty big mistake leaving home: We'd wheeled our luggage sets out of our garage with the pieces stacked and attached to each other so the house-to-house airport van driver could wheel them all down our short driveway to the shuttle first and then fit them into the car separately. But he'd taken them apart at the top of the driveway and carried them one by one to the shuttle—and when we got to the San Francisco airport, an hour from our home, we'd discovered that he had left one major piece in the driveway (between one of our parked cars and the garage, which is why we hadn't seen that it was still sitting there as we drove away from the house). We asked the driver if one of their other drivers could pick it up and bring it to the airport, especially if they were coming to the airport anyway, since that would take about an hour and we had two hours before our flight. The check-in desk said they'd let us put it on the plane as long as it was there about twenty minutes before the flight. But the driver refused to take any responsibility for the problem. We called his boss at Marin Door-to-Door, who also said, "Your fault."

Yes, we should have counted the bags—and you can be sure we do that now!

In the end, we called our house sitter and asked her to overnight the piece to us in Paris via FedEx. (We got her a bottle of her favorite European perfume to thank her; this was beyond the call of house sitting.)

We'd also gone shopping upon our arrival, to replace some of the essential items in the case, and bought one toiletry by mistake. We went back to the Paris department store, but they would not take it back unless I bought something else of the same value. They don't do refunds, even on a credit card. This sent us on quite a tour of the store, which involved going to three different counters: to return the merchandise and get a voucher, to pick out an item (nightgown), and then go to yet another place to pay for it with the voucher. This was at BHG, the biggest store in Paris, and I recommend the place for its vast selection of good-quality merchandise, but be certain that you want what you buy! And a day or two after we got to Paris, the suitcase arrived—to the airport, at least. But the Paris FedEx office didn't call me to tell me this; it was only after I called them several times that finally they had good news for me. Well, to start with, anyway.

At first, FedEx told me the suitcase would be delivered to our hotel. Then the next time I called, to find out when it would be delivered, they said they were missing some information. "What information is that?" I asked. They needed my passport and some other ID info, they said. I asked if I had to go to the FedEx office or if we could fax the copies. The fellow I talked with wasn't sure, and was in no hurry. *His* life necessities were not in my suitcase, clearly.

Finally, after a few calls back and forth, we faxed them the data, and they called to say it was illegible (at least they did call back), so we faxed it again—and finally, one afternoon after we'd been out having a good time, we walked into the hotel lobby and the receptionist, Beatrice, said, "Look who is here!" and pointed to my beloved peacock-blue suitcase (which has since gone to the suitcase graveyard, after ten years of travel).

All of which is to say: things of this nature do not go as efficiently in France as we are used to here in the US. (When a piece of our luggage went home with another traveler here, San Francisco Airport provided us with the name and phone number of the other person within a few hours, and the person brought our suitcase to us within a day. Another time, United rerouted a suitcase through the wrong city, and delivered it to us at home the next morning.)

Taxi, Please

Occasionally, French taxis will not take a fare that is less than about a half mile. I once got into a taxi in Paris at a stand near Notre Dame after standing in line for a bit, and when I told the driver where I needed to go (about four blocks), he refused to take me; he would not budge.

I was carrying shopping bags and had my cane. When I clumsily got out of the cab with all my gear, stunned, a young woman who was next in line at the stand leaned in to me.

"What happened?" she asked in English. "What did he say to you?"

"He told me that because I'm only going a short way"—I pointed off beyond Place de St. Michel—"only a few blocks, he would not take me. He refused to go."

She was kindly affronted for me and disdainful of the driver, in the way only a Parisienne can be, with pursed lips, a "tch, tch," and a shake of her pretty head. "They are not supposed to do that!" she said. "You should take his license number and report him."

But he was already down the road, and I let it go as one of the travel difficulties I sometimes encounter. The next taxi took me willingly, anyway, and I tipped him well.

We learned the hard way that if you want to get a Parisian taxi at a museum near closing time, that probably is not going to happen. The museum personnel are unlikely to be willing to call one for you. If you want a favor like that, ask at least a half hour before closing, but it still may be to no avail. Better to use your mobile and call one yourself. Restaurants, though, are always willing to call a cab for a departing patron.

At the Rodin Museum, five minutes before the gift shop's closing, I asked to use the disabled persons' restroom behind the gift shop (because the only other one was down some steep marble stairs, and there was no elevator). The museum itself was still open. The gift shop concierge told me no, even though I was using a cane, and she meant it. What a witch! Rather than risk the slippery stairs, I found a cab ten minutes later at the corner and rode another ten minutes back to the hotel—gritting my teeth in extreme discomfort all the while. So, allow yourself a good half hour before closing to use the facilities in France.

Not long ago, we went to the Musée d'Art Moderne on a rainy day and arrived in the mid-afternoon, feeling we'd have enough time to browse before it closed. We obtained a wheelchair from the nice concierge. (All museums in Paris have wheelchairs now, and if you have a walking difficulty, you cannot do a place like the Louvre without one, make no mistake. In fact, if you go to the Louvre—and you should—I recommend deciding on *one* section you'd like to see in one day. It is overwhelming and very tiring to try to see more than one period or type of art in one day there.) The personnel at the Musée required an ID as deposit for the wheelchair; they suggested my passport, but I decided I'd rather give them my driver's license.

When we were finished viewing the art (R. Crumb's interpretation of the Bible), we returned the chair— about ten minutes before closing. The two clerks on duty, however, could not find my driver's license in the small drawer in which they tossed all the IDs people surrendered to them.

At first, it looked like they were going to shrug and tell us they couldn't find it. They had definitely given up the search.

"Good thing I didn't give you my passport!" I said, with some cheek.

The clerk who was continuing the search did not find that amusing.

Finally, three of us, at my instigation, including the museum director, took everything out of the drawer and went through it bit by bit. As we did, I saw that the license was stuck along the side of the drawer, face to the wood, so the white back of the license made it nearly impossible to see against the white drawer.

Sigh of relief. They shoved the ID at me and then hurried us, me on crutches, down the slippery, wet, marble front steps.

"Do taxis come by here this time of day?" I asked in French. (This was pre–Lyft and Uber.)

"*O, non, non, Madame*," saith the door monitor *officiante* with her hand on my back, literally pushing me out the door.

"Then, would you please call us a taxi?" I asked.

"*O, non, non*, there is a taxi stand just near here." She pointed down the block.

We looked and, not seeing the blue taxi sign, I said, "But exactly how far?"

Did I mention that I was on crutches? It was quite obvious to her. And it was raining.

"It is very close," she said before slamming the door and locking it quickly.

I put up the hood on my raincoat and gingerly crutched down the slippery steps, and then Richard and I carefully set off on the wet sidewalk, with me placing my crutch tips slowly so they would not slip. We thought she meant that we could catch a taxi at the corner, but it was actually two long city blocks to the corner of a main street—and still we saw no taxi stand. Given the extra tension of caution in the rain, getting that far was exhausting for me, so we paused there, and I stood under an awning while Richard tried to flag down one of the many cabs that kept passing us by.

Eventually, a very kind taxi driver with a van full of passengers stopped, rolled down his window (despite the rain), and told us that no one was going to stop there because there was a taxi stand another two blocks away. Slowly, we walked/crutched the rest of the distance to the stand—where we got a cab immediately. We walked at least a quarter mile, probably more.

So I'm not a big fan of French bureaucracy, but, after all, they do seem to have invented it—it's their word originally. I think they kind of like things to be complicated. I like most of the French people I meet, particularly the hoteliers (okay, yes, they are being paid to be nice to me, but it feels genuine)—I just don't like the way a lot of things are run over there. Fortunately, the beauty of Paris makes all the cultural anomalies worthwhile.

Which brings me to a multi-cultural joke: In heaven, the chefs are French, the police are British, the lovers are Italian, the engineers are German, and everything is organized by the Swiss. In hell, the police are German, the engineers are Italian, the chefs are British, the lovers are Swiss, and everything is organized by the French.

There, I've offended just about everyone in western Europe. I didn't make up this joke, for the record, and it was originally told to me by my ex-husband, a foreign-car mechanic who hated working on Peugeots. And to be clear, the Parisian hotel we love, Parc St. Severin, has a very organized and accommodating staff, and I'm sure it's not the only exception to the blatant stereotype I've described above.

A Border Surprise

In 1982, when I left Israel with my group of companions, we ran into one serious problem. We had chartered a small bus for the eleven of us through a travel agent in Cairo, planning to return to Cairo since our long-before-purchased air tickets required flights from Cairo to either Europe or the United States. It was a comfortable, air-conditioned trip across the Sinai Peninsula to Jerusalem; however, when we returned to the Sinai border ten days later, we were informed that our passport visas were no good.

Upon entrance into Egypt at the airport several weeks before, I'd asked how long our visas were good and had been told "three months." But that was only if you didn't leave the country—a fact the soldier at the airport did not mention.

We were stuck for several hours in a cyclone-fenced, paved area with no seating between Israel and Sinai, while our tour guide unsuccessfully tried to negotiate our return to Cairo—kinda scary—until, after being told in no uncertain terms that we could not return to Egypt without new visas, Israel opened her arms and took us back.

We had to go to Tel Aviv for a couple of days and wait till the Egyptian embassy (also run by their military) was open (two hours on Tuesday, only) to get our new visas. This did give us time to enjoy the beach in Tel Aviv, and we single women enjoyed seeing the tall, handsome members of the visiting Yugoslavian basketball team wandering around town, so that was a plus.

So, there you have it: travel is fun and rewarding, but you should always allow yourself some leeway on timing, especially on flight days or at borders, and be flexible about other countries' rules and habits, which may seem strange . . . as ours likely do for many who visit the US.

PART 2:

My Mom Has Changed (or I Have!)

Taming the Wild Handicapper
(Unruffling Feathers)

———∘o◯o∘———

*A*ttitudes toward physical, mental, and emotional handicaps vary from hand-wringing and doting obsequiousness to compassionate acceptance of the disability as just another aspect of a person, to outright disdain. I'd like to think that last one is a result of fear, especially fear of how one would feel if the serious physical (or mental or emotional) limitation were one's own. Still, it has been surprising to me that some prominent figures have actually ridiculed disabled people in public, even in the twenty-first century, which shows little social compassion or awareness.

I was first inspired to write advice regarding how to be with a handicapped person several years ago, when I was talking with a woman acquaintance about aging and the difficulties of eventually becoming handicapped.

"Yes, I used to go to the mall with my mom every weekend," she told me. "Now, since she has trouble walking, she doesn't want to go anymore! I don't know what we can do together."

My first thought, which I did not express, was, *Put on your big girl pants and do whatever she wants to do. Take a movie to her house. Help her get in the car and go to a park and watch the birds. Sheesh.* But instead, I tactfully (and I am not always tactful) said, "It takes some adapting. You have to find new things to do that she enjoys." And then I gagged myself with a spoon. (Sorry.)

Actually, I get it. None of us is ever ready for that day when a parent ceases to be the rock of support or meticulous housekeeper or whatever they were before they hit That Point, which can come as late as ninety or as early as fifty. Dementia, of course, makes it more difficult to find things to do together, but even people with advanced Alzheimer's enjoy simple activities like listening to music, especially pieces they loved in years past. (If your Wild Handicapper is a polio survivor, I strongly recommend a booklet, *Post-Polio Health Care Considerations for Families & Friends*, published by Post-Polio Health International in Missouri. See my Resources section.)

Given that I am aware of a range of perspectives on "crip culture," I'm going to be so bold as to tell you here how handicapped people like to be treated, how they don't like to be treated, and what type of assistance, if any, they'd appreciate from you, their daughter or son, sister or brother, husband or wife, dear friend or caregiver. (By the way, the term here in the US is "caregiver," not "caretaker."

A caretaker watches over a piece of property. In the UK, as I mentioned earlier, those who assist disabled people are called "carers.")

Since my own limitations are primarily physical and are fairly serious, but not on the order of the severity of paraplegia, ambulatory difficulties are mostly what I'll talk about in the next few chapters. Obviously, I can't speak for everyone, so it's a bit arrogant that I'm about to attempt to do that. But I know enough people with disabilities or handicaps that I'm going to not only tell you my own preferences but also make some generalizations and attempt to point out some possible ways of being with us/them. I assume that you want things to be as easy as possible, not only for the handicapper but also for yourself. Most of us crips want it to be as easy as possible for you, too.

New Difficulties vs. Prior Conditions

It does make a difference whether a person has been disabled or handicapped for many years or whether it's a new condition. It has been necessary for me to live with partial paralysis and weakness for seventy years and counting. Sometimes it really pisses me off that it is so freaking difficult, or that I have new weakness or more severe fatigue than I used to have, or that my step falters more than it used to. I don't think of myself as elderly (though I am now seventy-three)—just as an older woman. Most friends in my age group are having a little more limitation these days too, but they can still walk a few miles at the least, or even go on a hike of several miles in the mountains, as well as being able to stand up at parties for an hour or so and chat.

That amount of standing and walking has never been in my ability quiver, and now there's even less there. Naturally, this state is frustrating and disappointing. I imagine that the average healthy woman ten years older than I am feels about the same. But the difference between us is, I've had plenty of time to get used to it, and I do ultimately accept my condition, though it's hard to accept the new problems as they show up.

I have known many people who have been left with a new and difficult limitation, temporarily or permanently, after an injury or surgery—I'm talking about breaking a leg and being on crutches for months, or having a leg amputated, or developing MS (multiple sclerosis), or going through treatment for a life-threatening cancer or a seriously debilitating stroke. These sudden problems are perhaps harder to deal with, psychologically and emotionally, as a previously healthy, able-bodied adult, than they are for folks like me, who have had years to adapt to such challenges. One day you're hiking the Sierras or dancing salsa, and the next you're lying in a hospital bed, being told you'll never again be able do something you love—ski, bike, walk, whatever. It's a life-changing disappointment no one is equipped to face.

Incidentally, I'm not a big believer in "you'll never do [insert activity] again," though sometimes this is the truth and must be accepted. I strongly recommend getting a second opinion. I also believe that it's wise to follow recommendations in your rehabilitation. Being positive but realistic and, most of all, determined and disciplined can reap unexpected rewards. Miracles do happen, and doctors can only guess at outcomes.

When I learn that I am going to lose activities that are dear to my heart, it motivates me to find other things I *can* do. But this is not true for everyone, unfortunately. Some people are so depressed by a difficult change that they are unable to emerge from their negative emotions. If this is the case for your loved one, a lot of patience and compassion will be necessary, along with some special diversions, and maybe even some mood-altering drugs.

For those who suffer an injury or illness that takes away a big part of their lives, there has to be a grieving process. Please allow for this, whether you are the Wild Handicapper or his or her caregiver, relative, friend, or lover. It is wretched to go through even a broken leg or a knee or hip replacement (especially a failed one; and knee replacements are the more painful and have the more difficult recovery of the two). The healing process can be quite slow, even for a person who does all the right things and has a basically sunny disposition, and especially for someone who's fifty, sixty, or older. Our immune systems and natural healing processes are just plain weaker in our senior years than when we were in our forties or younger.

Watch How You Say It

When your Wild Handicapper is suffering, it is not helpful to dole out aphorisms such as, "When God takes something away, He gives you something else"; "When one door closes, another opens"; "Count your blessings"; or "Be grateful for what you have; you get around pretty well!" For a person who's been dealing with physical limitation all of his or her life, those kinds of statements are irritating. After all, it's hard for a person who is not disabled to imagine how much of a daily grind it is, how wearing on one's energy, to have to constantly find solutions for worsening problems, compensate for things that can no longer be accomplished, or long for places that can no longer be visited as easily, or at all. Someone in this position has to do his or her own self-encouraging all the time, so the last thing needed is someone saying, "Think positive!" If the Handicapper comes up with the platitudes on their own, however, trying to summon up optimism and make it through these new challenges, certainly encourage that, at least at the beginning (and keep in mind that the "beginning" may last longer than you or the Handicapper thinks it should). A self-generated positive attitude is different than someone else repeatedly telling a person to look on the bright side. The helper's quiet (or not so quiet) confidence alone is the most helpful outside source of encouragement.

A note from my own life as a Wild Handicapper: although I have tried to eliminate a lot of sarcasm from my life and vocabulary (the original Latin meant "to strip off the flesh" and it still indicates contempt, derision, and ridicule), sometimes releasing anger with sarcastic humor can be helpful, as long as there is eventually an admission that I know what I'm doing: avoiding grief by stripping away the disturbing meat of the situation.

Creative Ways of Assisting

One helpful thing you might be able to do is bring over a comedy DVD and settle in for a good laugh with your friend or relative. Laughing at things that are happening to someone else whom we know is just acting, and expecting us to laugh at them, can be a great relief. Or tell your mom something funny that happened to you. Tell your dad about a mistake you made and how you made a fool of yourself. Laugh at yourself, and you might hear a story in return that on the surface is about a sad trip and fall but is in fact an opportunity for the person to find some humor in the incident.

It's possible, of course, that there won't be anything funny about the experience; sometimes we all just need to flat-out complain a bit. Just give your Wild Handicapper the space to do that. People often need to talk about their situation, not for sympathy but so the people who are close to them understand their limitations. That's intimacy: you learn things about one another that the public doesn't know, and it brings you together in a deeper way.

Venting occasionally isn't the same as spewing a constant litany of complaints, of course. That is really hard to listen to after a while and can become a bad habit. When I realize that's the problem, I generally try to shift the conversation to get the person's mind wrapped around something more positive. But that only really works if the person has had an opportunity to get the hard stuff off his or her chest. Therapy might be what's needed—which itself can present a problem, since older people tend to have a poor concept of what therapy is ("That's for crazy people!" or "I don't need some expensive professional to tell me what to think or how to be"). But especially when disability is new, it's great to have someone who is *paid* to listen to new, upsetting, possibly embarrassing assessments and attitudes about one's situation. And many counties offer free or low-cost mental health services.

My friend Leslie Scardigli, who eventually died of complications related to being paraplegic, once told me a story about himself and another paraplegic guy he used to hang out with. They were considering buying some real estate in Sonoma County so they could start an alternative educational facility (not related to disability but to fields such as yoga, arts, music, metaphysics, etc.). The day they went to see the property, they got someone to help them into one of their cars, which had adaptive hand controls, and then toss their wheelchairs in the backseat, and the two of them set off, excited about their independence and the prospect of getting out to look at a nice place in the country. They got to the real estate agency that had advertised the property and pulled up to the curb—and then looked at each other, realizing they were so used to having someone to assist them that they had not planned for getting out of the car. This was long before cell phones, in the late 1960s, and rather than lean on the horn until someone thought they were either obnoxious or in terrible trouble and came out to talk to them, they simply sat in the car and laughed until they had tears in their eyes. (Okay, they may have been smoking a little pot.) Then they turned around and went home. I love remembering Leslie telling this story around a candlelit table of friends, his dark brown eyes sparkling as he relived the absurdity.

Everyone has their own coping skills. Some people need to keep telling themselves things are going to be great—even if they are not—and some people need to go through a period of depression and grieving. (More on depression later.)

Of course, there's a point when you might need to say, "Okay, time to come with me to the park even though your face/foot/back is not what it used to be; I know it's hard, but you gotta do it sooner or later unless you plan to just sit here in the dark the rest of your life." (You may not want to be that flippant.) Or it may be time to say, "Mom, you've really been a trooper, but it's time to get a brace for this leg. The physical therapy has brought it as far as possible and the doctor's suggestion will help you be able to walk again."

Something like that.

The response may be a strong reaction. You may get some anger coming your way, or a torrent of tears you had not known was building up, or comments like, "You don't know how this feels!" You indeed may not, and it's good to admit that. But you may also be the one who has to bring up possible adaptations, if the Wild Handicapper has not yet accepted the change. Please try not to take the anger personally. Just listen. Be sympathetic. Put yourself in his or her shoes. You can even say, "I cannot know exactly what you are going through, but I think I would be really upset if it were me." Perhaps say something along the lines of, "I want to assist you to have the best life you can in your new circumstances. Help me out a little too, if you have any ideas about that. Whatever you want to try, if it's humanly possible for me, I will be here for you."

Now, not everyone is going to be ready for so deep a commitment. I don't blame you. Most of us have never wished to take up nursing as a hobby. And it's okay if you are not planning to be a caregiver; you can still be a friend. (Suggestions for "support lite" will be coming up later in this chapter.)

Be Patient and Keep the Faith

Your primary job as a caregiver or loved one is to practice a lot of patience and at least a modicum of optimism, as I've already implied. You may hate your Handicapper's attitude. She or he may drive you crazy. There is a balance to be found, and you have to put on your big-kid pants and be as mature as you can be, as loving and as sane as your best self always knew you could be, in order to find it. Richard has become good at this (most of the time). He went through a few years of not assisting me as much as I would have liked when I hurt myself, because he was afraid he would make it worse (a realistic fear). He was nervous about doing the wrong thing and also whether his efforts would be appreciated, especially after he tried to keep me from falling one time and my knee hit the pavement anyway and I injured myself rather badly.

I tend to fall somewhat frequently, due to my paralyzed foot and weak leg, despite my attempts to be careful, and in our early years together, Richard was frightened by my pain, fear, and anger when I injured myself or a new limitation reared its ugly head. It was hard for him not to be angry or frustrated about feeling helpless to make my situation better. This was particularly true if I were suddenly sitting on the floor in tears, worried about how bad the injury might be and not ready to engage in a rational discussion about what to do next. It has been consistently disappointing for me that I have many times not been able to make more serious injuries heal faster, or to stop using crutches and get back into the swing of things immediately. Each injury has been different.

It can be unpleasant to live with someone who has a chronic problem, or one that keeps repeating itself. *Not again* . . . may float through a Wild Handicapper's companion's mind, and it certainly is the phrase that comes up for me when I fall. When a spouse knows that there could be several weeks of difficulty and healing ahead (you never know when a fall occurs if it will be a two-hour recovery or a two-week or even two-month ordeal), it may be natural to withdraw a bit, unless they belong to the saintly few within whom the nurse gene predominates. Sometimes the specter of having to take on a few more tasks domestically or personally is deflating, particularly during a work crunch. It takes a conscious effort to be compassionate sometimes.

Now if Richard is home and hears me cry out in pain, and he is not lost in his own work, he often calls out, "You okay?" Just knowing that he's there and available, if I am not sure I can get up or have wrenched an elbow trying to catch myself before I go down, and having the reassurance of his care for a few minutes, is enough. If it's a bad injury, that's scary to both of us, but he's been through enough years with me that he knows that—probably—it's not the end of the world. In the first moments, it may mean that I need him to get my crutches or an ice pack, or, in rare, more serious cases, to give me a ride to urgent care for an x-ray.

Long-term injuries are challenging. I have had to be creative about taking care of myself after a bad fall. Cooking dinner is nearly impossible on underarm crutches, for instance, and I have a hard time even moving a microwaved dinner to the table when I'm using them—though I have done it. (In fact, I once did it while my roommate at the time sat at the table chatting and watching me do it without offering to help. I should have asked for help. But in these cases, I now spend a little money on takeout.)

Outside or Community Assistance

When I was going through breast cancer treatment, Richard and I found a service similar to a low-end caterer. They delivered meals once a week that came in a plastic tray that could be popped into the oven (but not a microwave, unfortunately). It was more expensive than a burger joint or groceries cooked at home, but cheaper than getting takeout at a mid-range chain restaurant a few nights a week, when I didn't feel up to cooking.

If your Wild Handicapper cannot cook and purchasing prepared meals is not an option, a rota of friends and relatives who can bring meals, at least periodically or temporarily, can be set up. Freezable stuff is really helpful, as is something that can be put into the microwave. Some communities have programs like Meals on Wheels that will deliver to people on Social Security. Some of them may be free. Then there will be at least one nutritious meal a day, or at least every other day. Check with a local food bank or Google "senior services" in the relevant area if this is something you'd like to address. Maybe a local church will have meal services, even if the WH is not a member; know, however, that some of these include proselytizing as one of their services (especially those missions "supporting" homeless people), something to which not everyone is interested in subjecting herself. Our county has an organization seniors can join for about $35 a month that provides volunteers who will do various tasks and errands for or even pay social calls to people who are disabled or can't get out.

These are examples of the kinds of things that will help out physically. Also, knowing that someone cares enough to set up a schedule and contact people will go a long way in letting a Wild Handicapper know that a loved one means it when he or she says they care and are doing what they can. No one can do everything (assuming there's no paid professional involved), and if there is no dementia involved, the WH *does* know this, regardless of behavior that may suggest the contrary. *AARP The Magazine*'s October/November 2015 issue even had a list of one hundred random acts of kindness one could do for a caregiver, nearly all of which were simple (and could, conversely and similarly, provide help or a smile for a disabled person).

Someone who is going through this for the first time, especially a senior, may well be disoriented by it and will need some help in finding creative solutions. It can be helpful to talk to an occupational therapist (OT). (They are not necessarily for people who work; in this context, "occupation" refers to learning how to do things in a new way if you have a physical problem.) One service OTs provide is to help people organize their homes and activities in a way that makes it easier to be independent and not hurt themselves. I went to one after I learned my swim program, and she opened up the world of better desk chairs for me.

I have recently enjoyed some OT coaching with regard to use of my crutches and my hands, which have become arthritic. It's good to check in with a physical therapist (PT) or OT every few years when one is handicapped, because new equipment or methods will have been developed that may make one's life easier. I had already picked up a lot of good ideas for more efficient living at home in Dr. Lauro Halstead's *Managing Post-Polio*—many of which are obvious, such as not fully making the bed each day, or keeping dishes and flatware as close to the table as possible. (The "keep it where you use it" rule.) It's relevant to non-polio disabilities as well. This book is especially easy to use because you can flip to specific chapters if you don't want to read it in its entirety. As to housekeeping, some of it will need to be ignored, unless you or your Wild Handicapper can hire a lot of help. My mom, who lived three hours away from me, balked at having even free help come in when she was aging; she insisted that she didn't need it, even though her home had become very dirty (her eyesight had become poor, and she apparently could not see—or smell—the grime). If you're facing a similar situation, you may have to bring the housecleaner one day and provide direction so Mom doesn't feel invaded or frightened.

In our county, there's a service called Whistlestop Wheels that picks up people who cannot drive to medical appointments. It costs about $2.50 per round-trip ride, and the rider has to be on Social Security. "Medical" is broadly defined; one of the members of my polio survivors' support group came to our meetings via Whistlestop. I also just heard about a program called Assist that gives people who are eighty or older round-trip rides to the store, a friend's home, or anywhere else desired for $5. These services drop off and come back to pick the person up later, so there is usually a wait; Mom will have to be patient and confident that the driver really is going to come back. (This may not be a great option for a big worrier or someone with advanced dementia.)

Setting Boundaries

As a caregiver, even an occasional one, it's necessary to take care of oneself as well. Part of that actually lies in being honest—both honestly kind (everyone I know can see through false or resentful "caring") and honest about what can be given and what cannot. Hopefully your Wild Handicapper knows you can't be there constantly (again, this will be a problem with someone with dementia; please consult with dementia-care people or read *The 48-Hour Day*, specifically written for family members of Alzheimer's patients). Statements like, "I cannot be here all the time. I am going to set things up for you so you can function when I'm not here, and I'll be back at six thirty/tomorrow/next week, etc.," are essential for people who have impaired cognitive function or those who feel especially vulnerable. Writing a schedule and posting it in a conspicuous place where it's seen daily will be necessary. Of course, people with advanced dementia should not live alone—something that may be difficult for both them and their family to accept, and to which adaptation must be made at some point.

My husband makes it clear when he cannot do things for me. I know what I need to set up for, and when I have his assistance and when I don't. He's matter-of-fact about it—though at times, when he feels bad about being unable to help, he may be short with me. People feel sad or even guilty when they cannot assist their loved ones to have the best life possible.

The other side of this partnership coin is that, as a Wild Handicapper, I have to remember to ask for what I need nicely, and I don't always. I am lucky to have a spouse who understands this. I am not saying it is always blissful around our house, but he at least knows that my frustration is something that does not last and is not related to him or what he has or has not done with regard to my disability, so he usually accepts my being that way. If I am too strident about my upsets (even if they have nothing to do with being handicapped!), of course, things generally don't go as well. There have been times when he's had to point out that I've been almost chronically angry for a couple of days. I'm definitely not the only one in the house who has anger, but taking a deep breath and attempting to be calm and solve the problem will always beat making excuses.

That said, I have read that at the time of an injury, swearing is actually physically helpful, particularly if there is pain. Something about it sets the system into alert mode, which reduces the pain and restores calm more quickly. (This is not an endorsement of long, drawn-out tirades, which almost always hurt anyone present, including the enraged person.)

Some people take advantage of the new situation of being disabled. This may hearken back to how we were raised. If Mama paid a lot more attention to us when we were sick (the opposite of my story), then having some condition that "allows" us to lie in bed and have people wait on us may be appealing. Sometimes someone who's been a mom or a wife all her life (or, more rarely, a single-parent dad) may think, *Well, it's my turn to be taken care of*, and be irritated if their lifelong caregiver role is not reciprocated when they need it. That's something to bear in mind. For others of us—and this is my own position—it's a situation we hate and hope that the worst of it is as temporary as possible. I am frustrated by not being able to get up and do and am a bit envious of people who can do nothing for long periods of time. In my life, that's what vacations are for.

Some people will really milk their unfortunate situation. I've known some myself. In the 1980s, I had a temporary housemate in her thirties who had a slightly painful hip or knee injury and started using a cane. It is my not-so-humble opinion that she didn't need the cane and used it to appear more debilitated than she was, which I thought was strange. She did not appear to be in that much pain, and even if she were, the point in using a cane would have been to use it until the injury healed and then get back to an active life, especially at such a young age.

One afternoon, we were in the kitchen together; I was fixing a cup of tea after work, and she had just washed a spoon with her fingers and a drop of dish soap (this always irritated me about her; she never fully washed her dishes, just kind of delicately did the minimum that could be considered "cleaning"). As I waited for my water to boil, she asked me, "Can you tell me how I can get on permanent disability?"

I was taken aback, until I realized that she thought because I had a disability, I'd know all about that. I was working full time and then some, but perhaps she thought I received disability income as well.

Regaining my composure, I asked her, "Why on earth would you want to be permanently disabled?"

"I just don't like working, and my hip and knee bother me. I'd like to quit my job because it would be easier for me. I figured you'd know how to do that."

I sighed. "Susan, you know, I've been handicapped all my life and have always worked; sometimes I work sixty hours a week. I don't think *I* would qualify for disability, even with a paralyzed leg, because I am able to work at a desk. Since you are able to do that as well, I doubt that the government would want to support you. You also would probably end up with less income than you get from working. But you could check with Social Security, if you are really serious, and ask them about applying for Supplemental Security Income. I don't know what the process would be, but I would imagine you'd have to get a letter from at least one doctor certifying that you're totally unable to work."

That was all I could guess about the process. I'd signed up for food stamps twice in the early 1970s, when my first husband and I were out of work, and each time it had taken two hours of waiting and a long set of very intrusive and humiliating questions just to obtain $50 in stamps. I decided right then that public assistance was too much work, and that anyone who applied for it must be truly desperate. I know there are people (mostly political conservatives) who think it's easier to find a way to be disabled than to try to be productive. So far from true—whether that mindset resides within those who don't believe in financial assistance for those in difficulty or those who, like my housemate did, want to find a way to take advantage of a temporary injury and stop being active—a choice that's almost guaranteed to push a person into actual disability.

But that is just one personality type. If your Wild Handicapper is like this, try not to get too wrapped up in it. Help him meet his basic needs if he cannot do it himself. If you find out he can do more than he says he can, cut back on your services, unless you think it's fun to wait on that person. (There are some people who are so sweet, funny, or entertaining that we may deem it a privilege to get to spend time with them, despite the work that may be involved. I'm not that person yet, but hopefully I can become that entertaining before I die!) You can also say something like, "I'll do this part while you fold the pillowcases." Sometimes working with someone is fun, and it's having to do things alone that makes it harder to get motivated. Or there's the incentive treat: "We'll watch [insert a movie name or stand-up comedy special, or some other fun activity, here] after you do your exercises and hang up your clothes." (Moms have used this technique for centuries. Now adult kids get to parent their parents.) Keep in mind that if personal tasks are always taken care of by someone else, hygiene especially, there may come a time when the person either cannot do these things or forgets how. Repetition of essential tasks is healthy and reinforces memory. It may take patience to wait while the WH does certain tasks, but it's necessary in fostering independence.

As to my former housemate, Susan, I have to admit that I really don't know how much pain she was in. It didn't appear that she was suffering much, but it's a dangerous road to second-guess someone else's pain level or degree of discomfort. I just thought she should at least try to find a solution for her pain, if possible, before going on the dole. But who knows, she may have had early arthritis and been in need of a joint replacement. Sorry for judging you, Susan.

Move It or Lose It

Another unfortunate thing that happens frequently with handicapped people is depression. This can lead to a lot of detrimental behaviors and outcomes. One of them is drug or alcohol abuse, particularly if a lot of pain is present. Another is lying in bed and wasting away, losing muscle strength. Another is just plain lying; sometimes people who have disabilities don't want you to know about things they do that they probably shouldn't be doing—for example, not taking their medication. Lying is an unfortunate but common behavior, one most likely born of shame.

Everyone needs to get oxygen running through his or her system on a regular basis. If your Wild Handicapper is bed-ridden, get her mobile in whatever way is possible. Maybe do exercises with the person—in a chair, in a pool, in the bed, or on the floor (assuming they have maintained enough muscle strength to get up and down from the floor—which, by the way, is a fairly important aspect of later life, as it enables getting up from after a fall). A wonderful gift, especially if you cannot be there as often as you'd like, is to send in a masseuse or physical therapist from time to time.

Movement is good for both the physical and the emotional heart. It generates optimism, especially if, over time, the person begins to feel a little stronger. Psychological therapy is also helpful, especially the method called cognitive behavioral therapy, but it's expensive—and according to a British study published in *The Lancet* in 2016, behavioral activation therapy is just as effective. This involves engaging in activities that have been appealing in the past, such as volunteering, reading, or spending time with friends. Again, some encouragement may be necessary here.

⌒∾⌒

Losing function feels so unfair, but it happens to almost everyone at some point. At first, it's easy to be in denial. Your friend or mom might say, for example, "I don't need a cane," when really the issue is how it looks—she feels that "only the elderly" use canes. It's natural to want to be seen as young and vibrant and able. But there usually comes a time when your mom, or spouse, or even you will need to admit that a little or a lot of assistance is needed. Chastising (even judgmental self-talk) is guaranteed to be of no use and will surely be detrimental, and ignoring the problem will exacerbate it—so my advice is to adapt to the changes the person you love is undergoing, as well as to your own body's changes. As we age, a primary trait we are called upon to develop is patience. Above all be kind—to your Wild Handicapper and to yourself.

Pain (Squawk!)

————∘o◯o∘————

Pain is a very complex process the nervous system evolved in order to tell us that something is wrong. Not nearly enough is known about this system, despite the fact that doctors, physical therapists, and neurologists have been studying it for decades—if not centuries.

Communicating pain is the brain's alarm system. However, after being in pain for a significant amount of time, the body tends to keep telling us we're in pain even when danger is no longer present, and we get into the habit of pain. That's not to imply that it's not real. It's real. Often too real. But rehabilitation of an injured part (or whatever has brought on the pain) can be difficult *because* of pain; if you need to exercise something to strengthen or recondition it and it hurts too much for you to do that, then of course a vicious cycle can set in.

Pain is relative. For someone who has not had much if any physical (or emotional) pain prior to the disability, any pain may seem unbearable. I have dealt with pain for

141

most of my adult life, but I am certainly not "used to it." I seem to have a lower pain threshold than a lot of people do, which may come with a generally sensitive neurological system. I do find, however, that I can often just power through it, until it gets to the point of my being unable to move, and then I have to stop and ice my back or spend a few days not doing much, or whatever seems to help.

Drugs and More

Someone who has endured a lot of pain throughout life may have found methods of coping, including a drug or exercise regimen that gives at least some relief. But drugs have their drawbacks—namely, side effects. I don't know of a single drug protocol that is fully satisfactory and renders a person pain-free while allowing them to remain fully alert and functional. I'm told that medical marijuana is helpful, but I personally don't care for being stoned anymore. I have been looking into using the tinctures or edibles that have a low inclusion of psychotropic chemicals (tetrahydrocannabinol, or THC) and only contain cannabidiol (CBD). I am told they relieve pain without the high, but so far have not found one in a cream form that works for me.

One thing I know about anti-inflammatories is that they work more efficiently if they are constantly in the system. You don't want to take them only when the pain gets bad—a practice often referred to as "chasing the pain." The ebb and flow of pain when it reaches a crescendo is an energy drain, besides being (duh) painful. Additionally, if a doctor *has* prescribed anti-inflammatories, I've been told by reputable physical therapists that it's possible to take ibuprofen at somewhat high doses several times a day for at least six months without risking liver or kidney damage. (Reminder: I'm not a medical professional! Check with your doctor about dosage.) That, of course, is only relevant if the injury is temporary.

I have been taking meloxicam, the generic form of Mobic, for several years. At prescription dosage, it's not a pain killer but an anti-inflammatory (inflammation is part of what causes pain, if not a major part), and reputedly it is slightly less detrimental to the liver and kidneys than ibuprofen. I also use Voltaren diclofenac gel on painful joints. I get a blood test to check my liver and kidney numbers once a year and have been told that it might be better to get the tests more often. The lab also tests for C-reactive protein, which indicates inflammation. Unfortunately, as of 2016, non-steroidal anti-inflammatories (NSAIDs, including ibuprofen and aspirin) were discovered to increase the risk of heart disease, so I'm trying to get off the NSAIDs— thus my interest in medical marijuana. NSAIDs are fine temporarily, it seems, but are not a good lifetime solution. Acetaminophen is not an NSAID, but it does absolutely nothing for my pain, and taken too often over several months or more, is also very detrimental to the liver. It is useful to some people, however, especially when combined with an opioid. I found when I took Percocet after a shoulder surgery that ibuprofen helped more for the pain, because the pain reliever in Percocet or hydrocodone is actually acetaminophen; the opioid is just a relaxant, at least for me. So I was still in pain but also sad—that's why they're called "downers." Not my cup of tea. A nurse recently told me that alternating acetaminophen with ibuprofen daily as a pain regimen can be highly effective. So that's another thing that could be tried—but again, only temporarily.

I am sympathetic to those who turn to drugs or alcohol because of their pain, though I do not support their use more than lightly. I hate to see addiction and its results, at the extreme end of the spectrum, but wanting to escape from pain, and the emotional and mental anguish or fatigue it can cause, is understandable. And if the person is very elderly, he or she may have made a conscious choice to drown the suffering, since they don't have much time left and even a year of severe pain is hardly time well spent. Of course, not being sober increases the possibility of falling or other accidents. But if you're sitting down, it can be fun to be slightly loopy. (Slightly, mind you.)

I want to make it clear again that I'm not condoning alcoholism or drug abuse (I support getting into a twelve-step program if appropriate). I am just saying I understand what makes people who are in pain, or have severe disabilities, turn to these "solutions" to annihilate the constant suffering. Life can be hard, and as someone who's known a few difficulties myself, I have a lot of empathy for those with severe disabilities and/or pain issues. I feel that a Wild Handicapper should not be treated as a sinner or laggard if they've fallen into this mode of thinking and behavior.

I have been told that you can't get addicted to pain killers, nor do they get you "high" if you are really in pain, but I've known people firsthand (a woman in my 2004 breast cancer support group jumps to mind) who've had to take increasing amounts of prescription drugs just to be able to function without pain. That's addiction. And the current opioid addiction is now a national crisis, with overdoses at a level we didn't see even in the 1960s with what was then seen as a period of excessive drug use. In a 2015 interview with Terry Gross on the program *Fresh Air* on NPR, David Linden, a professor of neurology at Johns Hopkins University, refuted the no-high concept. He said that it is not true that when one is in pain, an opiate or similar pain killer will not produce euphoria. The drugs will simply not produce *as much* euphoria, he said, as they would if taken when the person was not in pain. In *Healthy Years*, published by UCLA Health, I have read that addiction is a result of a chemical reaction in a person's brain, not a result of lack of willpower. Opioid-induced hyperalgesia is a condition caused by over- or extended use, and paradoxically causes the patient to have more sensitivity to non-painful or painful stimuli alike. Seniors are especially vulnerable to this, since they may be taking multiple medications at once.

I do find that even when I am in acute pain, opiates produce what I suppose is euphoria, but I don't enjoy that feeling: my thought processes slow down and I become less coordinated, which puts me at higher risk for falling—a much less pleasant sensation than the slightly giddy feeling induced by a glass of champagne. Some people say of opiates, "You're still in pain, but you just don't care." The giddiness of hydrocodone can be fun for a while, maybe a couple of hours, but being on opioids makes me feel permanently stupid. Plus, they are constipating, a state I was unfamiliar with before taking them and found to be almost as bad as pain.

Other Forms of Pain Relief

I've read about several studies that indicate that people who meditate, especially using the technique called mindfulness, report feeling significantly less pain than other people, and that it is particularly helpful for people who are trying to reduce pain medication. (Mindfulness is simply focusing on the present and watching thoughts come and go with no emotional attachment. I have at times been able to have no thoughts at all when meditating.) Interestingly, the meditators' MRI results showed slightly more activity in the area of the brain associated with pain but less activity in the regions involved in emotion and memory; the researchers concluded that their subjects were experiencing the pain but not the unpleasantness of the sensation, because their brains managed to avoid identifying the sensation as painful. Given this, meditation definitely seems worth a try. (I have gotten out of the habit myself but intend to take it up again, both for turning my attention away from pain and also to bring me peace from the frustration of dealing with my many physical challenges.)

There are now many modes of treatment for acute pain, including physical therapy and managed drugs and natural supplements. These sometimes have either a mild or very beneficial result. I take curcumin (a capsicum or pepper derivative), boswellia, cherry extract, and some other things that are natural anti-inflammatories and also reputedly do not damage the stomach or liver. They are helpful, but not as dramatically so as NSAIDs. I've tried glucosamine and chondroitin for the arthritis in my thumbs, and they make no difference in my pain level (they do help some people, though perhaps only 10 percent of sufferers), though the chondroitin's shellfish base has made my hair a little thicker!

Though I take a lot of different supplements, I'm not sure they help a great deal. Since there are few double-blind studies on them, there's rarely any real proof of efficacy or non-efficacy. It's kind of like clapping your hands to keep the elephants away; I keep clapping, and there are no elephants, so it must be working. More directly put, there may be a psychological placebo effect. I do notice a difference if I don't take some of them. Ultimately, one's money is probably best spent on a healthy diet and exercise.

A year ago, a serious rotator cuff tear and the subsequent shoulder surgery I mentioned earlier, followed by severe and debilitating irritation and weakness from a manipulative massage given by a licensed physical therapist, put me into the "Sorry, but there are some degrees of pain that are nearly impossible to tolerate" state. I was not able to move my arm more than a couple of inches after the botched treatment without feeling ready to burn down a house.

Before the manipulation treatment, I had been driving and on my way to normal functioning, slowly and carefully; I was doing everything I was told to do; my healing had been right on track. But then things got totally derailed. The physical therapist apologized, and the orthopedic surgeon gave me a cortisone shot, but I had to have a second one before my considerable pain was eased enough to resume physical therapy and rehabilitation, after more than a month of crying out in pain several times a day. (Despite decades of occasional physical therapy, I'd never had this experience previously. I consider it a fluke, caused by overzealous enthusiasm that the PT had because I'd been improving; she really dug in there!)

With any injury, I am constantly bringing myself back to "This too will pass." Perhaps it's naïve, but I tend to believe there are solutions for every problem other than terminal illness. I vacillated between anger, grief, resignation, and determination for many months after my necessary shoulder surgery. After I was released from physical therapy, having accomplished about 40 percent recovery and having been told, "You're in so much pain, Francine, that we don't know what to do about it and can't give you any more exercises until you are in less pain," I saw a body worker who practices Active Release Technique (ART) for several months. Now I am doing much better and have at least 90 percent of my range of motion back, though some movements still spark some pain. This is two years post-surgery.

It usually takes a year to recover from shoulder surgery, I've been told by a doctor friend, but in the case of a patient who is sixty or older, the time period is close to eighteen months. I was probably right on schedule, as frustrating as that felt. My surgeon says I will still improve but possibly won't regain the full range of motion I enjoyed before surgery. I'm not giving up, though!

Twelve-Stepping It

There are twelve-step programs out there if your Wild Handicapper gets a bit *too* wild. I know that many people are afraid of "The God Factor," but as a person who went through Co-Dependents Anonymous and Adult Children of Alcoholics for my relationship issues and misconceptions, I can attest that you can substitute "Inner Guidance," "Inner Peace," "Higher Self," or other terms for "God." The point is for us to give up thinking that we can control life, other people, our alcohol or drug intake, or anything else. It's helpful to accept that things just happen, not always for a reason, and that it's how we deal with them that makes life difficult or easy.

For some people, a rehab or residential treatment program may be the solution. But a recent Stanford University and Harvard Medical School review of twenty-seven studies involving nearly 11,000 participants did find that Alcoholics Anonymous was the most successful form of treatment for alcohol addiction, especially in terms of higher rates of continuous sobriety. I am not saying that participating in such a program is easy or quick or that all people will be willing to do this kind of work. But these maladies *do* have solutions, and a twelve-step program is one of them.

Physical pain may be what leads people to abuse alcohol or drugs. But underlying addiction, there is usually emotional pain that makes people want to annihilate their feelings. The twelve-step process and other programs can help get to the bottom of issues people don't even realize they have. When I did an inventory of traits I had that were not serving me, I saw that many of them, such as expecting people to know what I was thinking, came from learning my mother's codependency habits. It was freeing to learn to identify what was driving some of my negative responses to life; I felt like I suddenly had a blank canvas upon which to design new attitudes.

Pain-Induced Depression and Trauma

I am fully sympathetic to those who seek out assisted suicide near end of life, or who have thoughts of this as a way out of suffering, though one would hope that some solution might be found that would make life bearable. I'm bringing this up because I understand how difficult it can be to imagine a reason to want to live when you are in excruciating pain. Veterans of wars know this—plus they have the added trauma of having seen and perhaps done things no human should have to endure.

Speaking of veterans: There are myriad therapies available for post-traumatic stress disorder (PTSD) and depression. Currently, there is a movement away from calling PTSD a disorder, because the hyper-vigilance we experience when we are in danger is a natural and self-preserving response. Generally, from what I have read, the most effective PTSD treatment is psychotherapy with EMDR (eye movement desensitization and reprocessing, which does not erase the memories but does make them less triggering). The downside of EMDR is that the government does not pay for as many treatments as a veteran (or other patient on government-paid medical insurance) needs. So if this something you're looking into, be sure to check your health insurance policy to see how many sessions for treatment of depression or PTSD it will cover. There are therapists who will work pro bono and nonprofit organizations that support therapy for those who need it. A generous thing you can do for someone with PTSD is to find how he or she can get some help, make the appointment, take the person in your car, bring a book and wait. And possibly pay for the treatment if the sufferer cannot.

Sebastian Junger, a war correspondent, said in 2015 that the thing veterans with PTSD need most is to get back in a group with other veterans, where they feel safe and known. Our body system rewards us (with oxytocin) for contributing to our tribe through self-sacrifice; we have not evolved beyond this natural response. It's part of being a human descended from a hominid. And all types of trauma—child abuse, rape, serious injury, crippling disease—can cause varying degrees of PTSD. My grandmother was accurate in comparing me, when I was a child, to a soldier; I *had* been through a type of war, the one I fought to remain standing. Again, I heartily endorse support groups, psychotherapy, appropriate medication, and finding other constructive ways to divert one's attention from pain or stress.

About twenty-five years ago, I had lumbar pain that was so persistent and severe when I lived alone that I could barely crawl to the bathroom, which was only a few steps away from my bedroom, without crying or even scream-ing. After being on underarm crutches for a month with a broken knee, this resultant back pain was far worse than the knee pain. I was so frightened, frustrated, and agonized. At that time, I thought, *How many months, or how many years, could I endure this before I would seek a way out? I don't want to live on pain killers the rest of my life; I hate the woozy sensation. What kind of life would it be to lie in bed on morphine, Percocet, or Hydrocodone for years or even months—assuming a doctor would even put me on one of those prescriptions? No, thanks.*

I could not envision myself as a person who could only watch movies and read books, never got out of the house, and was constantly drugged. I respect those who have learned to live that way, however, and I know that value, and even purpose, can be found in any situation. One can, for instance, write, or scrapbook, or volunteer from home by making phone calls or working on the internet. Maybe some make art. But it was very hard for me to see myself, the active person I've always been, with friends who are also quite active, leading a sedentary and mostly solitary life, in severe pain and whacked out on codeine or some stronger drug. I live with a lot of solitude, but in the instance of that broken knee and resultant back pain, I felt very threatened by the idea that my future might comprise leading a life of isolation and further-restricted mobility. This thought represented immense loss at that time, especially since I lived alone and had no financial access to assistance. (More is available when one is of Medicare age, but I was in my forties then.)

Fortunately, I did not have to find out how long I could endure feeling like my body had a wild animal in my spine that periodically bit me; that level of pain lasted for only about five or six weeks. But those weeks were hell, and the pain affected all aspects of my life and my ability to find any enjoyment in it. I was working, so I could only take ibuprofen, which did help, but not as much as an ice pack. For those several, long weeks, nothing completely alleviated the sharp, intense pain I was feeling.

That renewed shoulder pain I experienced earlier last year made me ask the same question—*How long can I take it?*—but fortunately, the cortisone shot kicked in and after a month or two, I had regained at least limited function.

Being There While Your Wild Handicapper "Goes through It"

If the person is bound and determined to stew in his or her own juices, there just is not much you can do. But be patient; if you just come and hang out, watch movies, play chess, or simply spend time with the person, you never know—a change may occur. My mom managed to put the brakes on her criticism of me when she was eighty, three years before she died. I never thought it would happen, but she made the choice. I was relieved that we were on cordial and even affectionate good terms when she passed.

The worst is when the Wild Handicapper gets mean. Understanding it and being compassionate can sometimes reduce the tendency. Sometimes after a real purging, a breakdown or a cathartic experience, a personality change for the better may ensue. Mostly, though, you only see that in movies. The nasty old uncle having a change of heart and becoming the sweetheart everyone hoped he'd be due to his niece's devoted care? Don't hold your breath. If it's an ingrained habit, all I can say is I'm sorry; it's probably here to stay. And I hope you can hire someone to assist the curmudgeon, because no one should have to endure a really nasty temperament without being paid. If you expect an inheritance, I'd check with your bad uncle's attorney before you put a lot of effort into helping out, if I were you. (Ha! Just kidding—the attorney can't tell you who the heirs are prior to death. The rest of what I just said, however—not kidding.)

While we're touching on the subject of hired care, you should know that if there is any money in the Wild Handicapper's account, it's going to be used up before any government agency will pay to bring someone in as often as might be needed. Nor will any government pay to place your loved one in a care home for more than a few weeks or two months, unless he or she is a veteran. I hope Pop or Grandpa saved his nickels. People have a lot of misconceptions about what Medicare pays for. You may have always said, "I'm not going to take care of Mom; she'll be in assisted living," but I suggest you look into all of this well in advance to assess the options. Assisted living is not paid for by Medicare or any insurance, to my knowledge, except possibly long-term care insurance, which is not the same as health insurance.

The most effective encouragement for getting someone out of bed, out of a wheelchair, or out of the house is to make a goal. Maybe the person will never ride a horse again, but that doesn't preclude their seeing a favorite grandchild ride in a horse show and experiencing pride in someone else's achievement. And as we covered extensively in the first part of this book, for most people a disability does not have to mean never traveling again; it just means that traveling will be more challenging than it was before. You might try renting an electric sit scooter (if you have a large vehicle or can get a collapsible model) or a push wheelchair for your Wild Handicapper for a fair or music festival and see how that goes. It simply is not necessary to give up on getting out.

Later, perhaps, your WH may move on to bigger things. You might say, "Now that you know you can enjoy getting around, I'd like to take you to [insert an enticing spot] for a weekend." Yes, it will be more work for you, but it will almost certainly help inspire more interest and joy in life in your WH, which can only make your relationship richer.

If a trip like that is just too much physical and monetary energy for you to give, don't worry about it. Just hanging out and offering your Wild Handicapper some conversation and compassion will also be appreciated.

༄

Please remember, too, this advice: It's always better to say, "I don't blame you for feeling sorry for yourself," than it is to say, "Stop feeling sorry for yourself." Validating what people are feeling is more effective than telling someone not to feel something. Patience is, again, required.

With that in mind, I invite you to explore with me things people say that, with a little introspection, could have been said differently or not at all. I call this using one's "chat regulator."

Nesting, Pecking, and Perching
with Your Wild Handicapper

⸺∘◦○◦∘⸺

I have to grit my teeth when a person leans over me when I'm in a wheelchair, talks to me as if I'm ninety years old, and says, "Are you okay, dear?" especially when they don't know me. This attitude is offensive to me and to many handicapped people. A well-meaning Filipina wheelchair attendant at San Francisco Airport once started calling me "Mommie." She said it was a term of respect for elders; apparently, she assumed because I was in a wheelchair, I was older than she was. She was actually about my age or older, so I didn't take well to the nickname. (More on wheelchair etiquette later.)

I prefer people to say things like, "Do you need a hand there?" or simply hold the door open when they see I have a cane, crutch, or two crutches. No need to make a big deal out of it; just act like I'm someone carrying two bags of groceries—common courtesy, which many people do demonstrate. Unfortunately, I have also frequently approached a glass door at a doctor's office with no hands free (each of them grasping a crutch, or one with a cane and the other with files, bags, or packages) and had no one get up to open it for me. Or the person walking out the door at Starbucks will let it slam in my face when I am two steps behind him, even though I have a cane or crutch in one hand and am pushing a computer case with the other. I am constantly amazed at these occurrences.

To their credit, I find that today's young people are the most considerate of all age groups, though at least half of others seem to be lost in their own world. Women in their fifties are a pretty helpful group as well, possibly because by that time they've had injuries themselves, or kids who have had them—or perhaps they have older parents who now need a little assistance and they've seen firsthand that using an assistive device means you could use a little human assistance as well.

Conditional Kindness

I've noticed that people are more likely to rush to help a person who looks like they are in their eighties or older, especially if they are bent over and moving slowly. I cannot walk very slowly because I can't leave my weight on my weak leg for more than one second or I'll fall over, but I also can't walk as fast as most people—which means I essentially have one speed, although on a particularly limpy day I am slower. I find that this pace tends to make people think I am managing better physically than I actually am.

I had a refreshing experience at the supermarket recently, when I was both exhausted and in a lot of pain. I vacated a line because I thought another checker was opening up, saw that I was mistaken, and went back to the first line.

The fellow who had taken my place looked at me and kindly asked, "Are you in a hurry? You can have your place back . . ."

Pleasantly surprised, I said, "Well, actually, I'm not in a hurry . . . but I can't stand up much longer."

He made a slight bow, held his palm out toward the check-out counter, and said, "Please, go ahead."

He happened to look like Bruce Willis, who is a gun-rights zealot, but clearly even if this were true of Grocery Store Guy, that doesn't preclude him from being a gentleman. And in fact, I had more groceries than he did, so his actions were particularly gracious. Good for me to have my concepts challenged.

Handicapped, but Not Helpless

Perhaps there are some little old great-grandmas who are recently into wheelchairs and like being waited upon who might just love it if you treat them as if they were helpless. You are going to have to experiment. My experience is that most people who are handicapped want to be as independent, productive, and contributory as possible. We also want people to use common sense and empathy. I cannot lift heavy objects, and at this point in my life, I cannot walk while carrying more than about ten pounds. As such, I deeply appreciate a simple "let me get that."

I don't, conversely, need someone to say, "You don't have to do that; you should ask me." The truth is, many of us hate to ask for help, because we have to do it a lot. We want to save up our Ask for Help chits for when it's imperative. So when other people simply pay attention and offer, even in instances when we can easily go it alone, we are grateful.

When I feel strong, I wheel one or two bags of groceries to the car myself, even when the clerks or some gentleman actually offer help. It feels good to be able to say honestly, "No, it's okay; I've got this."

Some people need a little sympathy, some need a lot, and some don't want any at all. What's not okay to bring up now may be okay in a couple of months. Sometimes people really need to talk about their experience. It can alleviate the difficulty. Asking a tentative question like, "How did this happen to you?" or saying something sensitive like, "I'll bet this has really changed your life," can open up a conversation. I like to tell people about my experience of polio, as difficult as it was. I have accepted it, or probably 95 percent accepted it, and can speak about the early days with some detachment now. (Regarding my current pain, I don't have so much detachment, but I save most of my complaining for my time alone or for my dear and compassionate husband. At least he also gets me at my best and most normal, which is most of the time.) The polio epidemic in the 1950s is a part of history that I know very well, and experiencing that disease and its residual effects has made me who I am. Many people have either forgotten the polio epidemic or never knew it happened, and talking about it gives me the added opportunity to broach the subject of vaccines.

I like it when people ask me what happened to me, frankly and politely, without a tone of voice that conveys pathos—comments like, "I cannot imagine what you've been through. You are a real trooper." Conversely, "Oh, I feel so sorry for you; I could never go through what you've been through," is not particularly uplifting. I don't think of myself as pathetic. Of course, people feel sorry that we are like this—that we do not have fully functional bodies—and we're not exactly chuffed about it either. That's okay. But it's not necessary to make a point of it. My thoughts after a comment like that are, *You could go through it if you had to; I did not have a choice. Whatever confronts us is what we go through. I'm no different. I could never have imagined going through it until I did*. I don't say those things. But I have said, more than once, "Everyone does what they must."

"I'm sorry you had to go through this" is more compassionate than "I feel sorry for you." Hugs are great, except if you're trying to give them to a person who doesn't like a lot of physical affection. I like hugs from people I know well and love, but don't particularly like to be hugged by people I just met, just like normies often feel. Hugs from a new acquaintance can feel like pity, even when they're well-intended. The feeling of "I'm glad this didn't happen to me" sometimes overshadows the outpouring of love, and it can almost end up feeling like the *hugger* is the one who needs to feel some love, because your disability is so disturbing to him or her. I understand that and am usually nice about it, but I'd still rather reserve my hugs for people I know well, regardless of who needs them or why.

It's all okay. People can't help what they feel any more than they can help what they think. It takes a lot of practice to control our thoughts and feelings; I think we don't actually control them so much as train ourselves not to think along particular lines. I know I can't help what I feel; *I can only control acting or not acting on my feelings.* All that stuff about "trust your gut" isn't always reliable. I sometimes say, "Pay attention to how you feel," but honestly, how we feel is often the result of repeated experiences, especially when we were young. (I will now step off my soapbox.)

As a short person who is now sometimes in a wheelchair or on a scooter, I hate to be patted on the head. I have always hated it, and people do it a lot when you are shorter than nearly all other adults. Some people may like it, but I find that unlikely. My sister told me when she was in her eighties, and in a wheelchair a lot, that she just hated being patted on the head or petted like a dog or cat, even if the person meant to be affectionate. It's akin to being treated like a child—as if it's cute to be diminutive, or a person of less power than a fully functioning, standing adult. Standing always conveys more power than sitting, unless you are royalty. Maybe we're over-sensitive, but I'm just saying how it is for us. Some people have been surprised when I've told them I get head pats when in a wheelchair or on a scooter. They can hardly believe someone would do that, but it really is common.

Imagine Yourself in Someone Else's Shoes (or Chair)

When you're with someone who cannot stand for long (or at all), and they're in a wheelchair or even just sitting in a regular chair, if you can, squat down to talk to the person with direct eye contact, or get a chair and sit next to your friend or new acquaintance. It is hard to look up at people constantly. I have gotten a sore neck from long conversations while seated—and I love long conversations—and although I rarely use a wheelchair, I do almost always sit when I go to parties. I try to scope out a high stool to sit on so I'm at the same level as standers, or sit in a grouping of chairs, but that's not always possible, and most everyone stands in social situations, so they can mill around from one conversation to another. Usually, I stand as long as I'm able and then take a break or invite someone to sit with me if I really wish to talk. Many times, I'm happy to just observe others at a gathering, too, but ideally conversations are best with both parties at the same eye level.

Waiting in line poses its own special issues. I've had people grumble when I've gone to the head of a line, say, at the post office (always a long one), the bank, or a ticket office. When people see someone with a cane or crutches, they are usually fine with the person going to the front of the line. However, many people do not understand that if you need some type of aid to walk, it is hard to stand up, sometimes even for more than a couple of minutes. If there's a chair or bench available—which there usually is not—I'll go to the last person in line and say, "I'm going to be behind you, but I'll sit here and watch the line, because I can't stand up for very long." People always seem to appreciate that, that I am not playing the "crip card." No one likes a line cutter, and when people have been waiting for twenty minutes and the line's moving slowly, patience and compassion even for handicapped people is going to wear thin. Rarely, maybe one time in twenty, the person at the front of the line will say, "Come up here in front"—and I will, but only after asking the others in line if it's okay. No one has ever said no. (But then, who would?)

It annoys me when I'm headed for a line when others are too and they rush ahead of me because they can—especially when it's clear we're all headed for the same place (a ticket window, usually). This happens a lot. Then, no one offers for me to go ahead when I arrive at the line—even though they know I arrived at the venue just before them, whether by a minute or a few minutes. This to me seems an obvious courtesy, given that it's impossible for me to rush and I'd have been further up the line if I weren't handicapped. I know there's no ill intent, but still. It's just one of those times when it's easy to feel that people think handicapped people should not expect the same opportunities as normies, which I have found is a common though unconscious attitude. I suppose I could say to one of the rushing lemmings, "Hey, would you save me a place behind you?" Maybe I'll try that if I ever have the presence of mind to do so.

Parking for Crips

Let's talk about parking.

First of all, let's dispose of the idea that there are "more Disabled Person (DP) spaces than anyone ever uses, and they take up spaces that able people need." I've had friends in San Francisco tell me, "DP spaces are all OVER the place! There are so many of them!"

Every time I want to say, "Find me one so I can keep it in my trunk."

I have been to a very few places where there are what I would consider the right number of DP spaces in SF. Sometimes there will be half enough DP spaces at a museum or concert venue. Usually there are, oh, a grand total of two—despite the fact that if you look around at any classical concert, half the heads have white hair. A good portion of those folks are handicapped or will be one day in the not-too-distant future, not to mention the few of us who always were.

Sometimes when I go to San Francisco, or even in Marin County, after driving around for a while, I just give up on finding a parking spot within my walking ability distance of the venue (usually this happens when I'm shopping or trying to pick up a prescription). If I've visited a friend in the city and think I'll stop to pick up a chai on the way home, if there's no parking for a block, I just skip it and drive home. Depending upon whether I am having a good day (a four-or-five-spaces-away day) or a painful and weak one (a by-the-door day), I might come back later on my shopping or errand trip, or just go home and forego completely whatever it was that I was hoping to do. When spaces available for grocery shopping are all out at the edge of the parking lot, that's completely unrealistic for me, since after shopping I will be pushing a heavy cart with one hand while using a crutch in the other. Even parking garages are often too many blocks away for me (and that's assuming I could pay the high price for parking in places like San Francisco to begin with). These days I often go with Richard or a friend who lets me out at the venue and then drives by himself to park in a garage. So, if there were "so many" DP spaces in SF, perhaps I'd drive to the city more often.

Another frustrating issue is that sometimes DP spaces are taken by early-bird wheelchair users who have a caregiver, relative, or friend assisting. They get pushed to the venue, while I park a block or more away and have to walk, stopping to rest against street signs, lampposts, or what have you two or three times along the way. A person who wheels their own chair, especially if it's not a power chair, certainly ought to be parking as close as possible, partly for their own safety; it's a little unsafe to cross a street, especially at night, in a power chair or scooter, as the low head height makes the wheeler hard to see. But I appreciate it when a person bringing a wheeler to a venue and pushing them in a chair takes one of the DP spots a little farther away. If it's level ground, and the handicapper weighs less than 250 pounds, pushing a wheelchair is not really taxing work, especially for a short distance. Folks who are still walking but having a hard time doing so need close parking as much as those who hand-propel their wheelchairs.

Some DP parking spots are larger so that people with vans and motorized chairs or scooters have room to get in and out of their vehicle. They sometimes have an extra space next to them, for getting the chair or scooter out. For those with a ramp that folds out on the side of their van, space is needed for both the ramp and exit room for the chair or scooter at the bottom. Recently, a shopper at Trader Joe's parked in that empty striped space and made it impossible for me to get back into my car. They announced this over the public address system, which I found a little embarrassing, but the errant parker never showed up. So I had to get into the passenger side of my small SUV and clamber over the seat and compartment between the seats in order to get to the driver's seat. I did leave the person a note on his or her windshield; I tried to be polite, something along the lines of, "Please don't park here; handicapped people need more room to get in and out of their cars, and this made it nearly impossible for me." But the driver may have thought, "Yeah, well, you managed."

It is unfortunate, but we crips are now in competition for close parking and also for easily accessible seating in concert venues and similar places, especially with baby boomers getting into the physically difficult years. (In *Not a Poster Child*, I mention that I've had older people come up to my car window and shout, "You're not supposed to park here!" That hasn't happened as much in the last few years; they are starting to think I am a peer. But just recently, when I parked in the DP space at the library, an older woman looked at me askance, walked back to the front of my car to see if I had DP plates, and waited to see if I had a "real" problem or assistive devices. When she saw my crutch, she smiled at me and walked on. A voluntary DP police person, like myself.

Among friends, it's practical and polite to talk about who should get the driveway parking space at the party and whether to carpool. Among people who do not know anything about each other, however, conversation about who has the "worst" disability may be merely an internal conversation involving a little dose of resentment, possibly containing the phrase, "I'll bet they can walk."

People sometimes park in a DP parking spot when they don't have a physical impairment that makes it difficult to walk. Maybe they are "just running in for a minute." I have driven around a parking lot for five or ten minutes because there were no spots close enough to the pharmacy for me to be able to walk without having to stop and rest, and then seen a young man who was pretty buff stride to a car parked in the DP spot—no placard, no DP plates on his car. Another time, I saw a lady with a placardless car full of Nordstrom and Macy's bags park in a DP zone and go into a nearby restaurant. I guess she wanted to park close so she could keep an eye on her purchases. I peeked into the car to make sure she didn't have a placard on the seat or the floor—when you use them a lot, they are always close at hand, and I at first thought she probably forgot to hang it on the rearview mirror—but when I couldn't find one, I called the police and reported her. (I do not know what happened after I reported her. If she had a placard, she would have been able to get out of the $270 ticket. I know that there are some invisible handicaps, such as chronic obstructive pulmonary disease (COPD) and heart disease. But if it's that bad, the person can go to a doctor, get a prescription for a placard, go to the darn Department of Motor Vehicles, and wade through the application process the rest of us had to withstand.)

If your mom has a caregiver, you may not know that she parks in the DP zone and then Mom sits in the car while the caregiver shops. I've gone to Whole Foods *so* many times and seen an ancient little lady sitting in the passenger seat of a car parked in the DP zone. Then a woman in her thirties or forties, fully physically able, comes out and loads up the trunk with the groceries, gets in the car, and drives away. Please ask your mother's caregiver if they do this. If they are also disabled, well, yeah, makes sense. Otherwise, that's inconsiderate. The caregiver does not need to park there if Mom's not going in the store. A DP placard is not a convenience for people who accompany a handicapped person, it's a *necessity* for those who are handicapped and actually have to get out of the car and go into a store to do an errand. I had a relative who used to use his dad's DP placard, and he was someone who was actually *supposed* to get a little extra exercise. He was not doing himself a favor. As with most issues around disability, whether it's your own, your spouse's, your parent's, or your friend's, parking is really just another situation where consideration, forethought, and organization are called for.

Collaboration and Compassion

Since Richard brings in most of our income, I do most of the cooking, plan the meals, do the shopping, plan the greater part of our vacations, pay the bills, reconcile our health insurance and doctor bills (lots of phone calls; don't you hate that?), do our taxes, do the laundry (he folds), manage many of the repairs, and do nearly all the gardening. He takes out the garbage, washes dishes, keeps the pool chemicals in balance, fixes most of the electronic devices, carries the luggage, does most of the driving, and performs several other household tasks, on top of currently working a grueling schedule. He is a great housemate, especially considering he grew up with a stay-at-home mom and live-in help and had to learn as an adult to chip in domestically. We have it worked out. Sometimes I get tired and ask him to go get takeout meals—and, rarely, when he's got too much to do, I fold the laundry.

Caregiving (and receiving) of any kind is a partnership and can be arranged in a way that makes you and your Wild Handicapper feel like you're both contributing. For instance, your bedridden mom may enjoy doing some internet research for you, or making some phone calls, or performing some other administrative task one can do from bed or the couch. If she tells great stories, ask her to tell family history stories, especially if you record them for others; that's a great way to help her contribute to your family or community, and allow her to feel appreciated and valuable. You could also help her go through her belongings and decide what to get rid of. (Expect some resistance to this idea.)

Get creative with this partnership.

A lot of handicapped people are surly, or at the very least irritable, about their condition and cannot be expected to be all-nicey all the time. That line of questioning that goes, "Why can't they just accept it and not be such a jackass about it?" is not particularly helpful. Find out what they think is funny and make sure they get a lot of it. Dark "crip" humor may be just the ticket. Or bring over a bottle of their favorite libation (assuming no addiction) and sit out on the back porch for a couple of hours talking about that trip you took way back when or watch a ridiculous movie. Good times can be had by all, and no one needs that more than your Wild Handicapper. I know it isn't easy when someone's in a bad mood, but isn't your WH worth the effort?

Above all, it's helpful when people remember that handicapped people have all the same desires, loves, discernments, intellectual capabilities (for the most part), and emotions that everyone else has. Just as people in their eighties say they feel like the same person they were at twenty-five, only in a more limited body, handicapped people feel all the emotions they have always felt. We are not pathetic creatures who want to be pitied; we are people who want to live the best possible life, just like normies, and are simply physically limited—as everyone is likely to be one day.

Managing Doctors

———◦◦○◦◦———

One thing I've found about having physical issues, especially in the last ten to twenty years, is that the medical profession has become more and more swamped with caseloads. I cannot expect my doctor to remember everything about my condition. If she or he does—wow, lucky me.

Even when my doctor cares about me and gives me good advice, however, I do need to take charge of my own care, and if you have a Wild Handicapper in your life who can't do this—whether it's your elderly mom or your single best friend who is overwhelmed by chemotherapy—you may need to pitch in. Either go to the medical visits at least some of the time, look at the prescriptions (possibly research them to see if there are conflicts: my mother-in-law was taking up to five drugs, prescribed by three different doctors, that were causing her to have tremors, to the extent that she could no longer get a fork to her mouth without spilling her food), and make sure her appointments are scheduled correctly—all of that—or hire a medical case manager to make sure the care she's receiving is what it should be. There are now companies, mostly small local ones, that specialize in this service.

Tracking Your Own Medical Info

When I had cancer, I bought a big accordion file. In it, I had sections for surgery, oncology, plastic surgeons (fortunately, it turned out I didn't need those last two), radiation, research, people's suggestions about doctors or diet (kept the helpful ones, threw out the irrelevant ones), complementary therapies, and more, and I took it with me to all the early planning meetings and the follow-up discussions. This made it so much easier to find the thing I had read about post-op care or whatever topic it was and discuss it with the relevant doctor when the time came to do so.

"Boy, you sure are organized," my surgeon said during one of our office visits.

"How else could you keep all this stuff straight?" I asked.

She shrugged and said, "A lot of people don't even take notes."

I could never have remembered everything—recommendations, what phone calls to make and procedures to follow—without some system of organization when I was going through that odyssey. And I was in my fifties then, when all of us are sharper than we are twenty or more years later.

Now I have a different folder for each medical subject—my feet, legs, hands, bone health, arthritis in general, hearing/ears, and all my other body parts and issues.

I also have a binder for medical information with predesigned sections for prescriptions, lab reports, and so on, as well as a section for business cards, which is especially helpful. Whenever I need to call a doctor, I have their cards all in one place, and I generally note the names of their medical assistants or office managers, because I've found that using the name of the person who will relay information to the doctor or whoever actually deals with the issue can be really helpful in expediting responses to phone calls. People respond better when I remember their names and treat them like someone I know rather than as "the secretary" or "the nurse."

I realize that my method is a little "old school," but I don't like being dependent upon a mobile phone for information (our land line at home is far more reliable; we basically have no cell service in our suburban neighborhood—too many hills), nor do I like to have to turn on the computer and wait for the screen to come up, and then scroll around in there, when I can just open a book and have the info I want in less than a minute.

From the perspective of the doctor, we do owe it to them to be organized when we go in for an appointment. Based on the reduced amount insurance is likely to be paying them, they have to diagnose and treat us in about ten or fifteen minutes per visit in order to keep their practice in the black. With this in mind, I always take a list of questions with me to my appointments and leave room to take notes when they answer. If there is a serious illness involved, I take my husband, both so that he knows the situation as well as I do and also because such conversations can be very upsetting and it's good to have a second pair of ears absorbing the information. When I had cancer, for instance, I went over the conversation and my notes with him after one appointment with my surgeon and we found we had some divergent opinions about what had been said. I used that information to call back and confirm what the facts were, or the recommendations, or the side effects, or the risk factors, and so on, and I ultimately felt better about my treatment experience as a result.

Advocating for Yourself

I discussed issues I ran into with how doctors spoke to me in *Not a Poster Child*, so you may want to look at that chapter ("Deal with It") for a more detailed exploration of this topic, but I will tell you here that many doctors say a lot of seemingly inconsiderate or insensitive things to patients. "Well, obviously, you can't exercise," one told me, when actually I exercise more than many of my friends. "Your breast is so badly damaged," another said after I had had two lumpectomies—which came as a surprise, since Richard and I thought the surgeon had done a great job and it looked pretty good, considering that about 25 percent of it had to be removed. An orthopedic surgeon suggested to me that I have the bone in my weak leg cut and the leg stretched (this is only done with children who are still growing) or that I have a piece of bone cut out of the strong leg, which could have resulted in eventual amputation if that surgery did not heal properly. Another orthopedist—a really good one—told me that it was a shame I cut down an antique cane so I could use it (apparently, he thought only tall people should be able to use beautiful old antique canes, unless they were made for a short person in the first place).

Those kinds of comments may seem unbelievable coming from a person who works with physical difficulties or diseases all day. But the fact is, these doctors don't necessarily know what it's like to *be* a person who's handicapped (or scarred). I try to gently educate them. I've said, "*Au contraire*, I exercise several hours a week!" and "I wish you would have put that differently; I don't think I look damaged" and "What will happen if the surgery you are suggesting doesn't work?" It's my body, after all. I can ask people, even professionals, to respect it. I have also said to some masseuses or physical therapists that I'd like to keep the conversation to a minimum as they work on me, because they tend to be a particularly chatty lot, and it's best that I pay attention to how my body feels throughout the treatment (remember that overzealous massage that landed me in a lot of pain?).

I told one doctor's assistant, when the orthopedist tried to cancel my appointment after I had waited, in considerable pain, for nearly two hours to see her, that my time was also valuable, and that I'd had to take a cab to see her because I was so injured that I couldn't drive. The assistant had just asked me to "come back next week," and I insisted that this doctor give me at least five minutes to look at my injury and make a recommendation. And she did. She was a little bothered, but she seemed to get that I was a professional person, too, and had interrupted my workday to see her.

I've switched doctors in cases where I've felt I was not getting good care or was dismayed by their attitude (although I'd rather have a top-notch cancer, heart, or orthopedic doctor who produces optimal results than someone who is nice, friendly, gentle, funny, or makes interesting conversation). This happened with one primary care doctor, a young woman, after I asked her to be sure not to put any speculative notes in my file, because at one time an insurance company had taken my former doctor's written comment, "possible hiatal hernia," to mean I actually had one—which was not the case at all; it was just indigestion and poor posture!— and my premium was raised as a result. I'd had a real challenge getting that out of my file and ultimately had to switch insurance companies. This young woman doctor told me she didn't deal with insurance, so she was not going to concern herself with my issues in that regard. I wrote her a letter (after finding a different doctor) and told her she'd *better* care about her patients' insurance issues, because those would make the difference between whether patients could stay with her or not; it was her income and my care that would make a partnership with insurance companies. (She, of course, did not reply.)

I have written to other doctors about unnecessary extreme pain I went through at their hands (during cancer treatment—not my surgeon but adjunct doctors), and they also did not reply. I think they were concerned about being sued if they admitted to their mistakes. (One of them apologized to my husband for causing me pain, but not to me.) I cc'd these letters to the hospital and nurses, though, and subsequently heard from the nurses that I had made an impression and my complaints would probably benefit other women in the future in terms of the care they received.

I have also left particular medical practices (eye doctors come to mind) because their staff members were so inefficient or nasty. I don't believe I should have to fight my way through a maze of people who don't talk to each other and/or are not nice to me in order to get the care I need, or even just to get an appointment. If I lived in a rural area with few medical providers, I'd probably put up with more grief, but I don't, so I don't have to.

Getting a Little Personal with a Professional

I try to stick with medical professionals who have the best reputations, especially among other doctors, and to always be ready to give them and their office personnel all the paperwork they need in order to facilitate their work. An attorney I trust once told me that asking an attorney for the best attorney in a particular field is far more likely to yield excellent legal advice than looking to Yelp for reviews. Professionals don't always have engaging personalities, and clients are sometimes upset because they didn't hear what they expected or hoped to, but people in the profession usually know who's the best. This is just as true for doctors. Your aunt may have had a good hip replacement ten years ago with Dr. Smith and thought he was cute, too, but it may be that Dr. Najafi is now known to be the best in your area, even though he doesn't talk much or joke around with you.

I send holiday cards to the medical professionals I feel the closest to, and if I happen to find out their birthdays, I send a card then, too. They are human beings, not just brainiacs, and they remember patients who remember them and make an attempt to make their job, keeping us healthy, easier. Although it's not necessary to "get as personal" as I've indicated above with all of them, I have found that after they ask me how I'm doing and I answer, if I ask how they're doing as well, and perhaps ask something like, "Did you take a vacation this summer?" or "How do you like working only four days now?" they respond as if we are partners working together rather than someone who only advises me. It lets the doctor know that I consider him or her to be a human being with a life outside the one that serves me. They may not have time for much chitchat, but being friendly also seems to open the door for discussions like, "I read this in *Harvard Women's Health Watch*; what do you think about it?"

❦

Medicine is an art, not a science. My breast cancer surgeon told me that sixteen years ago. She pointed out, "You and Richard are numbers people; you want to hear what the chances are in different outcomes, and I can give you those figures to help you make choices. But it's really trial and error." Medicine utilizes science to effect an outcome the doctor hopes will follow a previous pattern. And doctors feel bad when the surgery or the drug doesn't work. It's not always that the doctor made a mistake . . . but sometimes it is. At the end of the day, we just can't expect them to be infallible, which is why I am all for enrolling them into a working partnership.

How to Use

Assistive Devices

∘◦○◯○◦∘

*F*or every single piece of advice in this or any other chapter, please check with your health practitioner, primary care physician, or physical therapist before following my suggestions.

I say this with a touch of tongue in cheek, because, for example, I've had more than one doctor give me wrong advice about using a cane. If they have not worked closely with a physical therapist, they do not know what it is like to limp, or to have a limb for which strength cannot be regenerated (and a very small number of PTs also don't know this). Doctors often think you use the cane on the weak side, when in fact that causes you to lean into the shorter or weaker leg and limp much worse. But as a converse example of what I would normally think is good advice, I am a big promoter of eating a lot of veggies (see the losing weight section), but it's possible you are not supposed to eat particular vegetables (like broccoli, if you are taking Coumadin).

So, although I of course think I'm mostly right in this chapter, my advice may not be for everyone. I am not a medical professional, I'm a person with experience managing a lifelong disability. But a bit of common sense is in order. Only employ my advice if you have assurances from your own healthcare providers that it will be helpful and not harmful!

Underarm or Axillary Crutches

If you cannot put any weight on one or both feet due to an injury or any other condition, you need to use underarm or "axillary" crutches. With this type of crutch, all your weight is often on your hands, placed on the handles, unless you have at least one foot you can put down. These crutches require shoulder and arm strength (which is why young men with foot injuries do pretty well with them). The underarm pad at the top of the crutch is meant to rest on the side of your rib cage a few inches under your armpit. Even if you are walking on both feet and using the crutches only for partial support or to alleviate pain, the tops should rest on your rib cage. If you rest them under your armpits, you can seriously impede the functioning of your lymphatic system and circulation. When I see people, especially kids, using them right up in their armpits (and I frequently do), I want to stop them and give a lesson on how to use them correctly—just what they'd love from an old lady.

The crutch should be adjustable to a height that accommodates the pad being in this upper-rib position.

If it is too long, you will be at risk for falling, with the tips too far out to the sides of your body, and if it's too short, you will slump over and eventually get a backache. You should be able to stand up straight even while using crutches. Weight should be carried by your hands, arms, shoulders, and the sides of your rib cage. I strongly recommend buying a pair of gel-padded bicycle gloves to use with them, or your hands are going to get sore in addition to being tired. (The gloves also look cool and athletic.) I like the Giro brand best; they have the most padding and some also have little loops sewn on the outside of the fingers that make them easy to tug off. They tend to range from $25 to $45 a pair.

To walk, put the crutch(es) forward first and move the foot or feet after them. With plenty of upper body and/or arm strength, a person can probably go along at a good clip by swinging the feet and body forward. One does need to be careful, however, because when the user is unfamiliar with gravity's effect, a swing too far ahead of the crutches can result in landing on one's tush—or further injuring the injury. (Re-breaking a break can require corrective surgery, the last thing desired.) I recommend taking it slowly till it feels easy, and even then, be cautious.

Many people, especially women, have told me that they just cannot use underarm crutches; they feel far too vulnerable on them. Good balance is essential, it's true; and these days, a bent knee scooter may be the best option anyway, but only if the uninjured leg is strong enough to propel the user and also reliable enough to stop it quickly.

Crutch tips need to be checked often if you are using them constantly for more than a couple of weeks. If they begin to wear, they will malfunction like a bald tire and will slip on wet or slick surfaces. This was a surprise the first time it happened to me, and it can cause a fall, especially since you are putting so much weight on the crutch. For this reason, I avoid using crutches in the rain whenever possible, and slow down to a snail's pace when it's unavoidable.

Be careful going over grates with either canes or crutches. I have suddenly had my cane slip out from under me after I walked over a grate that pulled the tip right off. Soft ground, same thing—it's rather like the suction of mud pulling off a rain boot. Keep to hard, non-slippery surfaces or dry grass, level if possible, for best results. Definitely stay away from pathways covered by leaves and graveled walks as well, especially those on inclines.

Going up stairs: Put the crutches on the level where your foot is (or feet are), if you can put a foot down. Then slowly lift your healthy foot, or both feet, up to the next-higher step. Then bring the crutches up to the same step, move your foot or feet up to the next step, and repeat. Putting the crutches on the next step before you put your feet up is absolutely the wrong way to go; it can wrench your shoulders and is pretty close to impossible to do anyway. When people try to do this, they end up saying, "I can't do stairs on crutches." And they are right, in that no one can do stairs that way.

Climbing stairs on crutches is a very slow process. Swinging yourself may result in loss of balance. Leaning slightly forward into the steps when going up makes me feel more secure and decreases the chance of falling backward, which is the worst possible thing that can happen. I prefer to have someone standing behind me if possible, one step down, who can put his hand on my back if I start to falter backwards, even if I don't actually start to fall. Just having someone there makes me feel more calm and secure and thus less likely to lose my balance.

If you cannot put any weight on either foot, stairs will be impossible, and quite dangerous to attempt. If your injured leg is in a full-length cast, stairs will also be difficult as heck, because you really need to be able to bend and lift the injured leg to get up even a few steps. If any of this applies, skip the stairs, walk a little farther, and take the ramp or elevator. If that's not an option, you can also sit down and go up the stairs on your bottom, one step at a time, dragging the legs. However, you of course then have to be able to get back up again, which is pretty difficult with a cast unless the rest of your body parts are very strong. Worst-case scenario, it may be necessary to forego a location involving stairs till you can put weight on at least one foot.

For going down stairs, the opposite principle applies: the crutches precede you. Put the crutches down on the step you want to access, then carefully move your feet or foot down. You have to be even more careful going down, since gravity will pull you forward. Lean back just slightly, staying close to the handrail, just in case. You can use it to steady yourself if you do lose your balance, or to pull yourself up if you end up sitting on the stairs. In some cases, both going up or down, you may be able to use one crutch and hold on to the handrail, though this poses the problem of what to do with the other crutch. I've had luck with tossing the other one up or down the stairs a ways and then moving it again after catching up with it; you can also hold on to it with the hand that's using the crutch, but if you have small hands, as I do, this is challenging. Having fallen both up and down stairs, I can tell you that it is far worse to fall down them. In the downward direction, I like a strong, reliable person right in front of me, descending one step at a time. That way, I can put a free hand on his shoulder to steady myself as well, if necessary.

Ramps: Essentially the same as stairs, except that they can be deceptive. Put the crutches in front first going down a ramp, and your feet in front first going up, with the feet or crutches following. If you put your feet first going down, you are likely to fall or lose control of the crutches. They are longer than your legs when they are behind you. (Draw a picture and you'll see; it's plane geometry.) If you extend the crutches first going up, they will again suddenly appear to be longer and you will strain yourself going forward to meet them, as you would when going up stairs. So, crutches first going down a ramp, and feet first going up—the same as with stairs.

Crutches can be used as support for a leg or foot while seated by putting the underarm end on the floor and the bottom tip next to your hip. (Just put a napkin or something down under the padded end if the floor's dirty.) The handle then becomes a footrest—helpful if you need to elevate it, which is usually essential with an injury. I don't recommend laying crutches on a floor when standing, because bending over to pick them up is not easy, especially with your foot in a cast. Lean them on something very close by or put them on a nearby table. Don't let people talk you into having them across the room ("Here, do you want me to put those out of the way?"), or you'll be stuck where you are until someone else is available to hand the crutches to you. If you can hop on one foot this is not as much of an issue, but it's much better (and safer) not to be hopping across a room if you can avoid it.

Lofstrand/Canadian Crutches

If you can put weight on both feet, your doctor may prescribe Lofstrand (also called Canadian) crutches, which generally have a hinged, movable arm cuff shaped like a "C," with an opening through which to slip your forearm. They can be bought without a prescription at medical supply stores and online. They cost more than regular crutches ($100 or more per pair, new; they are sometimes available used, though not as often as the underarm type), so your insurance may not be willing to pay for them unless they are prescribed by a doctor.

This type of crutch is far more convenient because you can keep them on while standing still, leaving your hands free (your arms still in the cuffs), unlike underarm crutches. You can write a check or hand over a passport or ticket without having to lean the crutches on something or put them down on a table or floor.

There is no reason to procure Lofstrands if you cannot support your full weight on at least one foot, because they require more strength than underarm crutches if used for full weight bearing. There is no bracing the crutch against the rib cage. They are intended for use when both legs can bear *some* weight, and serve essentially as a balance aid or for back relief in the case of one leg being shorter than the other. When one leg is shorter (and especially if that leg is weak), the constant extreme shifting of weight one engages in as a result of that asymmetry usually causes the spinal discs to swell on one side or become pinched on the other, or the vertebrae to become worn on one side; shifting some of the work of supporting your body to arm-cuff crutches allows some relief. (These spinal changes can result in *canal stenosis*, narrowing of the spinal canal, which usually causes the nearest nerve to be pinched or aggravated.) Lofstrands allow your body to continue to work mostly as it's designed. I have, however, noticed that my legs, hips, and back have become weaker after using them frequently for a few years. (More on this topic later.)

With Lofstrand or Canadian crutches, nearly all your weight rests on your feet, with a little weight on your hands. This takes significant pressure off your back, especially if you are limping. I have seen people try to use them like underarm crutches, with all stress on the arms and shoulders—a use they are not intended for, and which will result in shoulder strain. Only the strongest of athletes would be able to successfully do this, and it would not be advisable even for them. You'll want to approach stairs and ramps in the same fashion as you would with underarm crutches; however, since you are supposed to be able to stand and put at least a little weight on the problem foot or feet with Lofstrands, you may be able to just hold on to a stair banister and carry the crutches in your other hand and go up one half step at a time, especially if you are not in much pain.

With this type of crutch, you walk with the left crutch forward at the same time as the right foot moves, in tandem (vice versa for the opposite foot, of course). I find that I am slower with Lofstrands than I am walking with a cane or no assistive device, but for extended walking, I am less tired than when walking with nothing or with a cane, and they provide more support. If you are going to walk for more than a few minutes, you will benefit from wearing the gel-padded bicycle gloves I mentioned before, which I have also found to be comfortable and helpful when riding my mobility scooter, which has handles like a bicycle or motorcycle.

The next-most-supportive device after Lofstrands is a walker, which I'll talk about later. These are less convenient, and heavier, but essential if balance is exceptionally bad, legs or hips are quite weak, or so much back or hip pain is present that you're unable to walk without the walker.

Canes

The cane is used on the stronger or less painful side. If your right leg is weak, shorter, or painful, for example, the cane goes on the left. You tend to lean into a cane or crutch, so if it's used on the weaker side, your limp will be worsened and you will also be less stable. This is contrary to what some doctors (or even physical therapists) may tell you, but if they tell you to use the cane on the weaker side, they are not knowledgeable about the use of canes. I'm sorry if this brings your doctor into question, but it's a fact. It is also a fact that many orthopedic doctors do not know as much about assistive devices as physical therapists do. They are two different professions: one diagnoses and performs surgery, and the other is the professional to whom one goes for rehabilitation.

The only instance where you would want to use a cane or crutch on your weak, painful side is if you were using two canes or crutches at the same time. If you need canes on both sides for pain or weakness, however, I recommend forearm crutches or a walker; you will feel more stable and experience less strain on your shoulders and arms. When I have a weak day, I use Lofstrands. I have used two canes, but that works only when I have just a few steps to take, not for walking from one end of the house to the other and certainly not for walking down the block. Walking sticks like hikers use would be a better choice than two canes in that case.

A cane is meant to be there for stability and balance. One uses it like a third leg, and it goes forward with the opposite leg. You actually are not supposed to lean very hard on a cane, though I admit to a strong lean! Because I have so much weakness from polio paralysis in my most affected leg, I need to use my cane or crutch to take the weight off that leg if I am walking more than perhaps one hundred feet (and even less distance than that, if I'm having a weak day). If you are really leaning hard on your cane, you probably should get a four-tip or quad cane or get yourself some Lofstrands.

Once you get used to a cane, you may feel somewhat jaunty. They are a great support. I can walk farther and longer with a cane than with I can with no assistive device and am faster on my feet with a cane than I am when unassisted or walking with Lofstrands.

A cane should be tall enough so that your hand rests on it comfortably with your arm slightly bent when you are not leaning on it. One source I've read says the grip (handle) of the cane should be even with the wrist when arms are at sides, and the forearms should be at a 15-degree angle when the hand is on the handle. My arms are long for my height, however, and I've found that I like the cane handle to be about two inches above my wrist when my arms are at my sides and I am wearing my shoes. These guidelines also assume consistent shoe heights, so if you wear higher heels sometimes (which is either brave or foolish; I don't wear heels!), you'll need at least a couple of canes.

When picking out a cane, just see how it feels. A too-tall cane will not be very supportive and will likely waver when you press down on it while walking. A too-short cane, like short crutches, will cause you to bend over or lean too far to one side and have poor posture—which, over time, will lead to a backache or hunched shoulders. Your arm should not be completely straight when using the cane; if it is, the cane is too short. No matter how attached you may be to a handsome cane, do not use it if it is the wrong height. Either get it modified or display it as an art piece till you are ready to give it away. (Canes are easily cut down at the bottom tip, but take off only a very little at a time. A half-inch may be plenty of height reduction.)

I've found that the most effective cane style is one with a lever-shaped handle shaped sort of like an L or a T, but with some curve to fit the hand, sometimes referred to as a Fritz handle. These were originally designed with arthritic hands in mind. I'll explain more about handle preferences in the following paragraphs. Try a few before buying, to see what the difference feels like. If you're short like I am, a problem you may encounter when shopping for canes is that they will all be too tall, and you will not be able to get a good sense of how they will feel when you are walking. But you can at least feel what the handles are like.

Derby handles have a modified, almost S-shaped contour—a basic L-shaped format with a curlicue on the end—and are my favorite. It is possible to get them with left or right orientation, called an anatomical handle, so that they fit your hand very well. (Unfortunately, most assistive device stores are unlikely to carry a Derby, and even less likely to offer both right- and left-hand options. I have always had to purchase mine online.)

Another nice thing about a curved Derby is that the curlicue at the end allows you to hang your cane over your arm so you can have your hands free for a few moments if necessary (which is also true of a traditional J-shaped handle, often referred to as a "J cane," or a "crook" handle, which often has a nearly full circle handle, like a candy cane). Derbys can also hang on hooks and chair backs, which is more difficult to accomplish with a straight L-shaped handle, a closed-circle handle, or even a J cane. There are gadgets you can clamp to the cane when you want to hang it on a table edge, but then you have to have strong, non-arthritic hands to squeeze the thing open enough to get it around the neck of the cane. And it's one more thing to weigh down a purse or pocket.

I prefer, rather than carrying something extra, to simply lean my cane against a corner or a chair—where either I or some other embarrassed person will often knock it over—or put it on a table, or on the floor, and then wipe the handle and shaft with a napkin when I pick it up to leave. My cane handles have lots of nicks from falling over, but I just don't worry about that anymore. One can see that my canes have been well used.

There are some canes that have a straighter L-shaped handle that is neither right- or left-handed (the Fritz), and they are the next best after Derbys, in my estimation. With these two types, you get the most surface area pressing against your palm, which gives you the most support and is the most comfortable for your hand.

The worst handle, in terms of comfort, is the rounded full-circle J or crook handle, because the least amount of surface is touching the palm of your hand (only the top of the circle), which means a lot of pressure on that one small area of the hand. I will concede that a J-cane could be a good choice if the handle were padded and perhaps if it were a four-tipped or quad cane, the most stable of single-stick supports.

When you climb stairs, put your stronger foot and the cane on the stair first and follow with your weaker leg—preferably one half step at a time, although one full step is doable if you have a lot of leg strength. When you go down stairs, I've read that we are supposed to lead with the weaker leg, but I am not sure that is always best. Try it with just one or two steps before you attempt a staircase. When possible, I like to have one hand on the handrail—preferably on the strong side, if I have the option—and the other hand on the cane (or crutch) on the weak side, which is the opposite of how I walk with a cane or crutch. This is because I am essentially using the handrail as a substitute for my cane; it's much more solid. If there is only a rail on one side, that means I may be supporting the wrong side for a few moments.

Sometimes I hand my sticks to my husband or a friend and use both rails, if the staircase is narrow enough, to help pull myself up the stairs, which is my fastest method. However, whether or not you can do this depends on where you are and what's going on with stair traffic. In the US, we climb or go down on the right, and in the UK, they use the left, just like on the roads. If there's no one coming, I have no compunction about using the "wrong" side; if someone shows up, they are usually younger or abler than I am and can just wait a moment or use the other side for a couple of steps. This may embarrass whomever you are with, but I have rarely noticed anyone seeming to be irritated by this approach when they've seen my struggle with the steps and that I am making an effort to get up or down as quickly as possible.

Walkers

I'm not an expert on walkers. I bought one and it sat in my den unused for a month, so I returned it to the medical supply store. If you are really unstable on your feet, I think they are essential. They are less work than crutches, but they are also rather heavy if you are small (I am) or weak (I am, kind of). But they are lighter than a scooter, for sure, so if you will be the one getting yours in and out of your car, they might be the better option for you. I can see that at some point I will likely need one; I think they are good for assisting when a cane or crutches do not seem like sufficient support or when one is recovering from an injury or surgery, or a stroke. Getting up and walking is preferable to doing too much sitting, so if a walker is what it takes, go for it.

You do need to stand up straight when you use a walker; the handles should be high enough that your arms are comfortable and not so low that you are hunching over the device. You should be as close as possible to the walker as you walk, not following along behind it. You control the walker; it should not control you. When you get up from a chair, use the muscles in your thighs if you can, or use chair arms or a table for support to help you get up; do *not* use the walker itself for this, ever, because it could roll away, and if you have a good grip on it you'll roll away uncontrollably right along with it and most likely fall.

Word to the wise: I have noticed, as has a polio survivor nurse I know, that using crutches to support myself when walking has gradually caused the thigh muscles in my weak leg and also my back and hip muscles on both sides to become weaker. It is now harder for me to walk shorter distances than it was a few years ago. My friend noticed this after using a walker for a year or so as well. We both think we began using these devices a little too often, too soon. It's always advisable to be in the best physical condition one can be and do what is possible to maintain or improve strength before and while making the decision to use assistive devices. I am in the process of doing new but careful core-strengthening exercises to correct core weakness and going back to cane use when possible to avoid overusing my crutches. (For polio survivors, as with MS patients and some others, strengthening has to be slow and moderate in order to avoid fatigue and overuse of muscles. We don't always get back strength that we have lost in overuse of musculature.) Due to my two-inch leg length difference, however, crutches are a major assist for my back, so using them less frequently is a trade-off in my case. If I have back pain, it's important for me to use them. But for little sprints, I'm using my cane, or just one crutch.

Any assistive device will make one's life easier but also may allow some muscles to work less hard and thus become weaker. If a person is sitting too much, on the other hand, using assistive devices may actually help him or her get stronger by getting up and walking. So, choosing when to use a walker or other assistive device has a balance point. Waiting too long may result in unnecessary pain and fatigue but being dependent upon sticks or a walker can also result in less strength, unless alternative strengthening exercise is employed.

Bathing Assistance

Handicapped or disabled people often care about their appearance as much as or more than normies. I find that when I do a quick errand and look less than well-turned-out, it's not unusual for people to stare and then look away. Another handicapped friend says this is her observation as well; we have a sense that we are perceived as "bag ladies" if we're in sweatpants and no makeup. So if you're assisting a friend or relative, please allow time for that person to take care of their seeming vanity and important hygiene. Mom still wants to look pretty.

If you've sustained an injury and have a cast on one leg, I highly recommend getting a small stool—preferably plastic, with non-slip feet—and placing it in your shower or tub, unless you already have a seat in there. Then put a large, leak-proof plastic bag over your cast; wrap a folded dish towel around the limb above the cast; and use a huge rubber band around the bag and cloth to close the top. The cloth helps to keep water from getting down into your cast. Medical supply companies now make a plastic cast cover especially for this purpose, which has a kind of double-bagged apparatus with a cloth top and Velcro closure. It's easier than the towel-and-rubber-band method, but the covers can only be used a few times, so they are also more expensive. I'll let you decide if the reduced hassle is worth the extra cost!

If you are using a shower, position yourself so you can put your foot/cast out of the way of the water stream. In a tub, you either sit down in the tub and put your foot up on the stool or sit on the stool and put your leg on the side of the tub. If you are big and have long legs, strong arms, and good balance, you may be able to lower yourself into the tub and put your leg on the side and then sit on the bottom of the tub. Otherwise, you will need to sit on the side of the tub and transfer yourself over to the stool, or have someone help you. If none of this is possible and you have a tub and not a separate shower, you'll probably have to settle for taking a "sponge" bath from a basin until that cast comes off. (Dry shampoo, which is available in drugstores and beauty supply stores, may be in order as well.)

Movable shower arms are great for this process. They are worth installing if this is going to be a long-term situation for you. You can also use a large plastic or metal cup, jug, or pitcher with a handle to pour water over yourself. Shower chairs, obtainable at medical supply stores, are a big help, and some non-profit organizations even offer used ones for free.

Take it all slowly. Having wet feet, hands, and hips makes you vulnerable. You don't want to break some other part just getting clean. You can always sponge bath till you have able-bodied help or become stronger—or, if this is a permanent condition, consider installing a walk-in or roll-in shower, or even moving to a home that already has one.

∽

Assistive devices do draw attention to walking difficulties. It is often the case that people think they will look "too old" or that people will think something else about them that is unflattering if they begin to use a cane, crutches, a walker, a wheelchair, or a mobility scooter. I have heard about this image issue repeatedly not only from children of aging parents but also from friends and spouses of those who may have a bad back, fallen arches, or worse: "He doesn't want to use a cane"; "She doesn't want to use a scooter; she thinks it makes her look old or lazy." These mobility aids may also bring up thoughts of "losing independence" or losing the appearance of ability or youth. But walking poorly for a long period of time will likely cause additional problems, and if a person uses a mirror to watch how he or she walks with or without a cane, for instance, it may be seen that the cane brings improvement to the way the walk looks (this happened to me with Lofstrand crutches and it was a hard fact to take in). Psychologically, it can be hard to accept that one really does need a device in order to walk better, save energy, or be safe.

I know I didn't want to use a scooter at first. Acceptance, though, has opened up my world. With my scooter, I can go much longer distances than I could when I was limping along on foot, only able to walk a block or two. I disembark, walk around a bit (for instance, at a park or museum), check things out, and then resume my ride. I now see and do far more than I used to. It's actually fun, and trying to do all that walking was not.

I say, embrace this change. Anything that keeps us moving better and longer is the way to go.

Staying Upright in
the Nest, Sweet Nest

————◦◦◯◦◦————

*H*ome is not only where the heart is; it is (ideally) also where one feels safest. The kind of flooring one has, what is on top of it, and how furniture, appliances, and belongings are arranged in the home will make all the difference in lessening falls, conserving energy, and increasing function over as many years as possible. It's possible to approach this with an eye to beauty as well, so no worries that I'm recommending going minimalist— unless that's the look you love, of course.

Making Your Home More Fall-proof

Small area rugs should be avoided, and when used, should have a non-slip pad underneath. The thicker or the lighter weight they are, the worse the trip or slip hazard. Nearly any area rug can be a trip hazard, particularly if one limb has no ankle motion (drop foot)—the effect of paralysis, a stroke or cut motor nerve from back surgery—as is the case with my foot and ankle. A drop foot's toes catch on things, whether with a shoe or without. When you trip, you may be able to catch yourself (hopefully not on a piece of furniture or a counter, as I have done more than once), but if you slip, you will almost always land on a hip or flat on your back, potentially hitting your head when you collide with the floor.

The older you get, the more likely it is that this balance challenge will occur—and increase in frequency, too. If you like area rugs, they all need to have non-slip pads, and even then you will need to take it slowly around the house. (I'm the worst offender on this front; I frequently run late and am in a hurry. I need to take my own advice, and not be hasty.)

Wall-to-wall carpeting is more dangerous than hardwood flooring, because shoes, especially tennis shoes or "trainers," with their grabby soles, catch on carpeting and lead to twisted ankles and knees. Tennies or crepe soles catch on flooring as well, especially glossy linoleum, but not as frequently or with as much grab as carpeting. Thick carpeting may feel cushy underfoot but it's a major hazard for twisting ankles or tripping. People with strong ankles and good balance may not notice this, so if your mom's balance is faltering, pay close attention to whether she has thick carpeting in her house when you visit. If it's time to replace, make the new rug as flat as possible—and even if it's not due for replacement, I advise pulling it up. If there's hardwood underneath, put in a large, low, heavy area rug instead of carpeting

(a safer and also a cleaner option, especially if anyone is allergic to dust or lint.)

Tile floors are disastrously dangerous; more serious injuries result on tile than on any other flooring. Water on a tile or marble floor is the slipperiest of all. And if you fall on a tile, varnished cement, or marble floor, you are much more likely to break a bone. (Senior women who break a hip, especially in their eighties or older, usually do not live more than two additional years because of the extended recovery period and lack of exercise following the injury. This is not something to take lightly.) Also, dishes break immediately when they hit a tile or cement floor, whereas on a wooden or linoleum floor they are more likely to bounce. Wood "gives" a little when an object (including a person) falls on it. That's why, when I hear a friend say she's putting in a tile floor, I try to dissuade her from it, especially since most of my friends are in their sixties or older.

Vinyl flooring can also be dangerously slippery, especially when wet. I have slipped and fallen on vinyl a lot (as well as on marble and tile). Old-fashioned porous linoleum is not as slippery, but it does need to be sealed (be sure to use a non-slip sealer).

Richard and I have hardwood floors and low, large area rugs for warmth and quiet in our house. We even have hardwood in the kitchen, and have found no problem with water damage; we just wipe it up when it spills. As long as your sink or dishwasher have no leaks to damage the floor (and possibly cause dry rot), wooden floors in the kitchen are safest. We have cocoa palm in our master bath, as it's less permeable to water. Bamboo is even more water resistant, but I wanted a dark floor and staining bamboo requires a thick—and extremely slippery—varnish. (I have found that our bathroom skylight has faded the dark cocoa palm, however.) If you like a blond floor, bamboo is a great, renewable resource choice for your kitchen or bathroom, but it's also a little harder than a hardwood such as oak, cherry, or maple, because multiple layers of thin bamboo are glued together for flooring. So bamboo is not as forgiving when you fall, or drop something breakable, on it.

We have no electrical cords trailing across from one point to another, especially around pathways; they are piled up under furniture or, in a couple of instances, strung under rugs, though this can be a trip hazard if the cord is thick. Same is true of those cord minders you can get at office supply stores; they are about a half-inch thick so can present a trip hazard in and of themselves (though not as bad as a cord, which can wrap around a foot and pull you down).

Stringing a cord across a floor is an invitation to catch a foot (especially a foot in a sandal), and down you'll go. We are also more prone to falling if we bump into something in a narrow passage, and may bruise or even break a body part if falling against furniture, so it's important to leave a lot of space between objects (like furniture) in your home. I also need some space for my sway back and forth due to my limp; my upper arms knock into knobs and edges when I don't have enough room, and walking sideways is difficult for me, so I like my passageways about two-and-a-half to three feet wide. We had all our doors widened (save one, from a powder room into a closet) when we remodeled our house two decades ago. This will facilitate any need I have for a walker or wheelchair in the future as well.

Young pets can be a problem, since they tend to run in front of you without warning. Mature pets are slower and more predictable (and often more in need of adoption!).

Planning for a Future Nest

While we're on the home front, the following is specifically for adult children with aging parents, but if you are an aging parent, aunt, or uncle, it won't hurt to read and consider these comments yourself.

I recently read an article at Money.com called "How to Talk to Your Parents about Moving Out of Their Big Beautiful House" in which the author, Penelope Wang, suggests that it's good to have a conversation with aging parents or other relatives about moving to a smaller more manageable home *before* they start losing cognitive ability and before there is a crisis. I agree. Most people want to remain in their homes for as long as possible, but that is not always realistic. Stairs, bathrooms on the second floor, steps upon entry, too much furniture for passage with canes and walkers, throw rugs, places (including yards) that are too big to maintain, and not enough money to pay for significant help are issues that can rear their heads earlier than you might expect. Ms. Wang says that rather than dictating to your parents what you think they should do, you should get involved in small ways to assist yourself in understanding their needs and finances. You can offer to help with bill paying or manage a home repair job, for instance. When you are more involved, parents are more willing to discuss more difficult topics, such as moving, wills, executor choices, and estate planning, even if the time frame for the change is still well into the future.

If you are the person who is aging in a place that may be difficult for you to manage in the future, I encourage you to begin to consider the advantages of an easier home. More free time and less worry may begin to appeal to you, more than nostalgia or the features of the home itself, sooner than you think. I am attached to my home as well, but I hope that if I get to the point where it's too much, I'll be able to kiss it good-bye fondly. I know this would feel like a loss, but I would not miss the maintenance, or the expense! I have had a wonderful life in my big ol' house, and someday it may be time to let a younger family enjoy it as much as I have.

Conserving Your Physical Energy

This is especially important—critical, in fact, for polio survivors and those with multiple sclerosis (MS) or chronic fatigue syndrome. There are books on this, and I recommend that you read at least one; *Managing Post-Polio*, by Lauro Halstead, MD, is my personal favorite, and is relevant to those with chronic fatigue or MS, as well. You can find more material on occupational therapy (not necessarily about work, but about how you use your tools and home, as I mentioned previously) and efficiency methods. Since I was an efficiency consultant for factories for a few years, these types of suggestions seem obvious to me, but for starters, consider the following.

If you live in a two-story house, either install a stair elevator or move to a single-story home. Stairs are the biggest possible physical drain for those who need to conserve energy. (Richard and I lived in a two-story house for five years, and after the first two years, I was more exhausted than I'd ever been in my life.) It takes literally ten times as much energy to traverse the same distance using stairs as one uses on a flat surface; that's why step aerobics and stair-training exercise machines help you lose weight. We looked into stair elevators in 2000, and I found a used one for $5,000. We decided that since we knew we were moving to a one-story home at some point, we didn't want to put bolts in the hardwood stairs of our 1939 vintage home, so I accelerated my search for a one-story place instead.

Don't make the bed every day. You have to walk around the bed once or twice if you're doing it on your own, and it's one more energy drain. Just pull the blankets up and call it good, unless company is coming.

Put things close to where you use them. For instance, your plates and silverware should be as close to where you eat as possible, especially since a stack of plates is heavy and will only feel heavier as you age.

Sit down to do food prep. If you have no low counters in your kitchen, either replace one with a low, bar-style counter or sit at a table to chop veggies (the dinner preparation activity which, I find, takes the most time).

Get rid of stuff you do not use or love. Stuff takes time and energy to maintain. (I am the worst offender, and again need to take my own advice on this!)

Park as close as possible to your destination. If you can't find a close parking space and the errand can be done on another day, go home or do something else instead, or have your spouse/a friend/a companion drop you off and park or run the errand for you.

Every time you go from one room to another, look to see what needs to be moved, such as papers, a sweater, or dishes, so you don't have to make an additional trip. If you have stairs, trip planning and organization is especially important as is getting a stair basket with a handle. We used to have one that was actually shaped for two steps on the bottom when we lived with two stories, and it was a useful time-saver for me. We left it when we sold the house, and the new owner (who, incidentally, wasn't handicapped) loved it.

Install or buy raised beds for gardening. (This is another area in which I'm shaking my finger at myself. We talked about them when we were designing our garden seventeen years ago but decided against it because I didn't think I'd need them only five or so years later; I had fantasies that gardening would not be difficult for me until I was at least in my late sixties, and that my husband was going to learn to love working in the garden. Ha!)

Eat lightly and get a little exercise; extra weight tires the body. Constant sitting gets too little oxygen into your system and also weakens your structure.

Now that you've got the picture, I'm sure you can think of a lot of things you can do to make your own life, or that of your aging parent or spouse, easier and safer. Start with something simple, such as giving away unnecessary area rugs or other trip hazards, or moving things around in the kitchen so that they're as close as possible to where they'll be used. And turn on some music while you rear-range things, too—make the changes fun!

How a Healthy Bird Behaves
(Plus, Tendon Pain and Rehab)

⸺∘O○O∘⸺

*Y*ou have probably been an adult for a long time, but I'm still going to offer you some pieces of advice, just like your mom or your doctor or your best friend would: my not-so-secret and simple—but not always easy, till you get into regular habits—ten clues to living a long and healthy life, assuming that's something you'd like to do. It can be daunting to tackle a lot of changes at once, so if there are several things on this list that you or your Wild Handicapper are not currently addressing, try changing just one thing. It might not be immediately apparent that this will improve a person's health or outlook, but just as it takes a seedling a long time to become a plant, these changes, even if they're slow to take root, will eventually bear fruit.

Okay, so here they are—my practical, and not magic, fixes:

1. Don't smoke tobacco.

2. Get at least two hours a week of exercise. Even if you cannot get out of bed or a wheelchair, you may be able to do some chair or bed yoga. (See my Resources and Bibliography.) If no form of exercise is possible for you, cut down on your calorie intake, especially simple carbohydrates.

3. Eat a balanced diet. Mediterranean is best for most people: a large variety of veggies, some whole grains, legumes (beans, lentils, etc.), some fruit, nuts, few simple carbs (limit sugar and anything containing refined white flour—this is the hardest part, in my estimation, but worth it; just have a treat once in a while and enjoy it), and maybe some fish or chicken and occasional meat. If you have digestive issues, you may need to alter this; talk to your doc or a licensed nutritionist. Add some mushrooms; they can greatly reduce memory issues, according to a 2019 Chinese study. And remember, diet is easier to control if you cook at home.

4. Brush your teeth at least three times a day (yes, three; I have been a two-time brusher for years but I'm mending my ways). A 2019 study I read about in *The Times* of the UK found that poor oral hygiene—i.e., brushing less than three or even four times a day—can allow bacteria to build up in your gums and seep into your bloodstream, leaving you with a much greater chance of heart disease. And you gotta floss, too. A dental hygienist once told me that if I didn't want to floss all my teeth daily, I should just choose which ones I wanted to lose and skip those. Sigh.

5. *Try to avoid stress, find ways to relax, and socialize.* If you can't sit still and meditate, then walk in nature or just around your neighborhood. Listen to classical music. Watch a comedy. Be sure to spend time with friends and/or relatives. A good social network is key to low stress and longevity.

6. *Get six to eight hours of sleep (on average) per night.* If you are sleeping more or less than that, you might want to check with your doctor. A short nap in the afternoon—just five minutes to an hour—once or twice a week is likely to reduce your chance of heart disease by nearly 50 percent, according to a 2019 Swiss study.

7. *Get all the vaccinations recommended* for your age and immune system.

8. *Wash your hands.* I do this every time I've come home. Contaminated surfaces— especially surfaces that have been touched many times by several people—often lead to illness, particularly colds and flu.

9. Get a full checkup once every year, or at least every two years. If you've had any major health issues or scares (high blood pressure, cancer, stroke, other heart disease, diabetes, cognitive problems), go in more than once a year.

10. Go easy on alcohol; not more than one drink per day (on *average*) for women, and one and a half to two daily maximum for men. Besides the dangers of alcoholism, heavy drinking can cause obesity and also cancer—and even one drink per day, for women, has a strong correlation with breast cancer.

Other than those ten tips, genes matter, and you can't do anything about those. But you have control over all of the above. I know it's probably all stuff you know already, but here it is, all in one place!

Of course, even if you have good genes, these ten life practices won't stave off all physical issues. The following pages are what I have learned about taking care of oneself specifically regarding tendon pain, which is something I've had to deal with frequently over the last decade or so, and I have learned that many aging folks have these same tendon problems.

Once again, always talk to your doctor or medical professional before implementing any of my advice.

Healing or Improving Tendinitis or Tendinosis

Not easy. When tendons are tight, they really hurt a lot. The nerves in the tendon sheath can send shooting pains that may feel electrical in nature, or as if someone has hammered the area. This may cause a stabbing pain that wakes you in the night. This is not something you want to live with, so it's better to work on the issue, as daunting as that may be.

First, get a referral from an orthopedist or your primary care physician to see a physical therapist. A good PT will have creative ways to—albeit very slowly—heal or improve your tendons and/or tendon sheaths. When tendon sheaths become inflamed, the condition is known as tenosynovitis, referring to the lubricating synovial fluid within the sheath. The tenosynovitis needs to be relieved before one can comfortably do exercises to heal the tendons contained in the sheath, but not all sore tendons also have sore sheaths. Using Kinesio tape will help relieve the sheath (more info on this follows below). Active Release Technique (ART) is also remarkably helpful for tendons. Google this term with "near me" (or your town) to find a practitioner, often a chiropractor who has been trained additionally in ART.

Tendons take months or even years to heal, especially when you are past middle age and beyond. Maintaining their health may have to become a permanent part of your daily routine, if you want to minimize pain and keep functioning. Perform the daily exercises and treatments you are given faithfully; don't give up!

I wrote an article called "Conquering Mysterious Foot Pain," about alleviating the pain of tendinitis or tendinosis usually caused by fallen arches, in 2009 for *Post-Polio Health International Newsletter* (see Resources for link). It contains a series of exercises that, if you have a "flat foot" that is causing you pain, you may want to try. Also, shoes with a tight strap across the top of the foot can be the cause of tendon pain. The exercises are simple, and doing any of them will assist you. Doing all of them will take about fifteen minutes a day when you've worked up to the maximum. It may take a few months of work, but foot tendon pain can be lessened or even healed— and the relief that effort brings is well worth the endeavor. I recently had a recurrence of tenosynovitis and tendinosis in my strong foot and did these exercises and the taping routine again, ever hopeful for recovery. After a few months of doing half as many repetitions as I should do, I had some improvement, and gradually the pain went away. This condition may recur again, but it's reassuring for me that I know how to alleviate it with dedicated exercises.

When nerve pain in my foot gets so bad that it wakes me at night—a very rare occurrence—I take an extra 100 mg of Neurontin/Gabapentin. This drug is helpful in very small doses (300 mg or less), but I found it caused headaches when I got up to 700 mg a day. The pain doctor I had been seeing at the time wanted me to work up to 1500 mg or more a day for my back and arthritis pain— but besides the headaches, at that level, a side effect can be suicidal thoughts, the last thing I needed. So I take 200 mg before retiring (to alleviate the spasms and pain a post-polio patient can have during sleep) and the extra

100 mg if I'm having rare, sharp, unrelieved, wake-me-up nerve pain in my foot.

The healing process will generally include icing the sore area (see the back pain section below regarding ice packs), getting ultrasound treatments (these have not helped me at all but are very helpful for some people), laser light treatment (really effective for me), taping with Kinesio tape (if your PT knows nothing about it, ask him or her to take a course on this—or find a different PT), taping lightly with Coban tape, alternating ice and heat, and, most importantly, doing exercises to stretch and strengthen the tendons.

As my orthopedist told me, tendons love to be stretched. A pulled muscle needs to rest, but it's rare for a tendon to get overstretched or torn except in a serious injury. They are more frequently under- or over-worked. Often, with a sore tendon or pulled muscle, the affected tissue may have been weak to begin with. That is why, for instance, the arch of the foot may become flat instead of retaining its form, which is critical to the supporting architecture of the entire body. That arch is actually holding you up, just like an arch under an ancient stone bridge. (I don't mean to say you're ancient, but if the shoe fits . . .) The muscles or tendons surrounding the inflamed tissue will need to be strengthened to support the weaker parts while they heal. It's a little tricky, but by paying close attention, it is possible to discern whether you are using one muscle or tendon or the one next to it.

Tape Assists

Coban tape is much better than a regular ACE bandage for wrapping a foot, ankle, or wrist. (I have found that it does not work well for a knee, for which a lightweight bracing support can be purchased and will also serve better than an ACE bandage, which, to be effective, has to be wrapped too tightly around a knee to be comfortable and to also allow good circulation.) Coban can be taken off carefully and reused a few times. You cannot wash and re-wear it repeatedly like you can an ACE bandage, but it is very thin and fits under shoes and sleeves easily.

When wrapping with Coban, stretch it to its maximum first, and then wind around the affected part with only a 25 percent stretch. It should not be tight. You also do not need a long bandage, as you might with an ACE; two or three times around may do the work of supporting without cutting off circulation, and the traditional figure-eight application is not always necessary.

Avoid the small cylindrical elastic slip-on arch bandages sometimes prescribed for fallen arches; they inhibit circulation.

Kinesio tape is a fantastic innovation! It has adhesive on one side, and it gently pulls the deeper skin away from the muscle or tendon so that it can gain better circulation. This "skin pull" is something the wearer doesn't notice— you just feel the support of the tape—but it really makes a difference. I have sensitive skin, and the adhesive used in this tape does not irritate as even a Band-Aid can (except if the Kinesio tape is pulled off right after it's applied in order to start over; you can't reapply it once it's been applied, and the adhesive is strongest when you first press it on).

I found that with the tendon issues I had from a fallen arch, wearing Kinesio tape for a few weeks alleviated my tenosynovitis irritation enough to be able to do strengthening exercises. I had not been able to do the exercises when I first went to the physical therapist, because they were further irritating the tendon sheath. I have also used Kinesio tape on a hamstring-related injury, on my rotator cuff tendon injury, and during post-surgery recovery, all with excellent success. Do remember to be patient, though. Rehabilitation of tendons is much slower than muscles or bones and can take months to a couple of years.

On my strong sore foot with its fallen arch, the PT started the Kinesio tape on the outside of my knee, with two inches at the top unstretched, as an anchor; ran it down next to my shin bone; made a sharp right turn across the top of my foot (the sore tendon), stretching the outer edge of the curve so the tape didn't crease; ran the tape under my arch; and then anchored it again with two unstretched inches under my foot near the outside. No matter where you apply it, the first and last two inches of the tape should *not* be stretched so they can act as anchors at each end of the strip. The calf muscle and foot tendon indirectly support the foot's arch, and the tape gives additional help.

For a painful tendinosis in my upper thigh/bottom at the ischial tuberosity ("sit bone") area, the tendon connecting the hip and thigh bones, we ran the Kinesio tape down from the spot at the bottom of my butt to a couple of inches above the back of my knee, close to the inside. I dealt with this pain and oversensitivity for a few years, as tendinosis is permanent damage (as opposed to tendinitis, which is temporary), but can now say that I have had a couple of years at a time with little or no pain in that area. It is stable, as long as I do not bend over too much for too long (which happens when I garden for more than a half hour, for example) or sit on hard surfaces with no cushion for more than a few minutes. I bring a cushion everywhere I go now, in case a restaurant, a park, or a friend's home has unpadded seats (as does a doctor friend who has the same problem).

My experience is that Kinesio tape reduces pain by at least 25 percent and assists greatly in healing over time.

❧

I know it's hard to keep up all the many things we must do in order to stay mobile and in good health. Perhaps it will make you feel better to know that you are not alone; there are about 73 to 77 million baby boomers in the United States as of 2019—roughly 23 percent of the population. So it at least shouldn't be hard to find a friend with whom to partner for exercise and good health encouragement!

Care and Feeding of
the Wild Handicapper

⋯⋯⋯⋯⋯∘◦○◦∘⋯⋯⋯⋯⋯

*Y*ou or your beloved Wild Handicapper may have already figured out all the ways of taking care of the body that are workable for you/them; it's different for everyone. But if not, here come lots of tips!

Back Pain

I experience back pain almost daily. Sometimes it's so bad that I cry and swear and become a very unpleasant person. This has been true for about a decade, but I've learned how to handle it (for the most part), and I also promised myself when this issue started to nag me that I would do anything I could to avoid back surgery.

Back pain is not simple. This is a section that really requires you to know what your particular back problem is, so definitely get some professional advice, preferably from a physical therapist. However, a lot of what I'm suggesting is fairly simple, *probably* won't make things worse (again, check with a professional!), and may help you.

If your back pain is debilitating but caused by something relatively minor, such as slightly swollen or wedge-shaped discs, minor arthritis, or canal stenosis (narrowing of the spinal canal) that is not advanced, I'm about to share some stretches and exercises that have helped me counter those same issues with great success. (For a quick and immediate fix, I find that an ice pack is best, and I'll talk about that later in this chapter.)

Yoga and Core Strengthening

Core (the torso muscles below shoulders and above thighs) strengthening is essential for almost everyone, but for people with paralysis or one shorter leg (and possibly those with chronic fatigue or MS), it is the key to preserving the ability to stand up, both on a day-to-day basis and over a lifespan. That said, definitely make sure it's okay for you to do yoga before you try these exercises.

There are lots of books, pamphlets, and videos on beginner or even handicapped persons' yoga. I learned my first yoga moves in my twenties, from some book I can no longer find in my collection, and from a few classes. Some senior centers have classes on chair yoga, and some older yoga teachers offer this as part of their curriculum. Be sure to tell the teacher about your limitations. I have a DVD that even includes bed yoga for those who are bedridden, either temporarily or permanently—but for the exercises I do, which I'm going to describe in the following pages, you have to be able to get down on the floor and get back up again! If you can't, you may want to watch a show like *Sit and Be Fit* on PBS or Youtube (a DVD of this program is also available), or find a different DVD on chair yoga, or check out local classes. (See Resources for links.)

Sometimes we are more likely to take up a regimen and stick with it when we have buddies to share it with or a course to which we've committed ourselves. The members of my polio survivors' group greatly enjoyed doing chair yoga at one of our meetings and also found that it energized them.

According to the *AARP Bulletin*, one study found that women who did yoga regularly had five times less inflammation than those who were beginners or did it only occasionally. Inflammation is the cause of many diseases and conditions which deteriorate our health. But doing even just one yoga stretch daily is likely to improve how your body feels, especially after a few weeks. And as yoga teacher Eugenia Esquivel, a rheumatoid arthritis patient, said in *Arthritis Today* in 2019, "Focus on what you can do, not on what you can't do. Don't compare yourself to others."

What you'll need

I find yoga mats really helpful—they keep you from slipping around as you might on a hard floor, and don't irritate the skin as rugs can. I prefer to roll one out on a rug rather than a hard floor; my slightly arthritic knees, hands, wrists, and feet hurt less when I push into light padding on the floor while doing my poses. If you think you cannot afford a mat, I got one for about $8 at a Ross store, and yoga teachers will also sometimes give away their old ones, which still work just fine. (Just take it home and hose it off in the back yard if possible, or sponge it off and hang over a chair outside to dry out.)

I've worn a nightgown, even with a robe, to do yoga, but it's really better to put on some sweatpants, leggings, or stretchy shorts and a top that doesn't flop around a lot, as sometimes the edges of loose clothing get caught on body parts or under the body, inhibiting a stretch or movement. Jeans are not going to be stretchy enough, and it's also not comfortable to wear a bra unless it doesn't have underwires and is very stretchy. Sports bras are apparently helpful for some women.

Adapting to your own individual needs

If you can get down on the floor, you need to be able to get up again, so make sure you can do that first. My method for getting up is to get on my hands and knees, then straighten my legs and arms like a monkey, then put my left forearm on my strong left thigh and stand up from there. I figured out how to do this by necessity and was later told by a chiropractor that putting your forearm on your thigh above your knee when you bend over is a suggested form for saving your back (I admit it—I was proud of myself!). You can also get down on the floor by holding on to a solid heavy coffee table or chair for support, and furniture can assist in getting back up again as well.

Getting up and down from the floor is really something everyone should have a method for accomplishing. As we age, we're more likely to trip, slip, and fall, and you definitely want to be able to get up from a fall on your own, if possible.

Generally, you want to breathe out when you exert yourself, and also when you bend forward in any pose. It's not necessary or even good to hold your breath; keep breathing in a normal rhythm.

Most yoga teachers start with a standing stretch with arms overhead, "greeting the sun," and then bend down, either touching the shins with the flats of hands or putting the palms flat on the floor, if the body is that flexible. The pose reached by "walking" the hands forward with the heels kept on the floor so that the backs of the legs get a good stretch is called a Downward Dog (I think it looks more like the monkey walk) and is often the next movement before lowering oneself all the way to the floor. I decided to forego this movement for a few years because of wrist pain but am now able to do it again without pain, so I'm carefully re-adding it to my routine. As an alternative to Downward Dog, I like to sit up straight with my legs out in front of me, grasp my feet, keeping my back straight, and hold for a few seconds to get a hamstring stretch.

Exercises for Back Pain Relief, Core Strengthening, and General Body Wellness

These stretches and movements have a natural sequence that flows easily from one to the next when done in the order I've described here. There's no obligation to follow this order, though, if you find a different sequence works better for you.

In any yoga or core-strengthening pose, you want to breathe deeply throughout your practice, imagining the breath going down into your abdomen.

My usual first move helps to relieve low back and hip nerve pain, including sciatica.

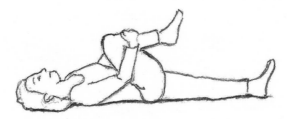

Figure 1

Lie down on the floor on your back and pull one knee up to your chest, holding across the shin, with the other leg straight on the floor, and hold for twenty to forty seconds *(Figure 1)*. Then straighten that leg and pull the other knee up and hold.

Next, embrace both shins and hold your knees to your chest for the same amount of time *(Figure 2)*.

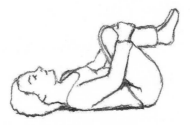

Figure 2

Without lowering your legs, turn your knees to one side and lower them to the floor, shoulders still flat on the floor, and spread your arms out straight *(Figure 3)*. Hold this position for twenty to forty seconds. You should feel a stretch not only in the hip on top but also in your shoulder, if you are doing this correctly.

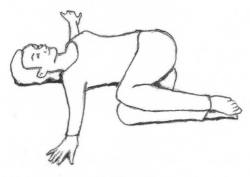

Figure 3

The last movement in this first set of forms is to stretch the top leg out straight, up and diagonally to the opposite side, with your foot reaching your outstretched hand, and hold *(Figure 4)*.

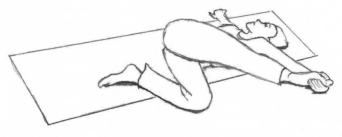

Figure 4

You may not be able to reach your foot all the way to your hand to start with, but over time you may gain more flexibility, as is true for nearly all yoga positions. After holding for twenty to forty seconds, bend the leg again, rotate your knees to the opposite side, and repeat Figures 3 and 4.

I have found that when I am having low-back nerve pain that radiates out to my hip or goes down my buttock to my thigh (sciatica), these stretches really help to alleviate it. Between each exercise, I press my low back to the floor, pulling in my belly button, and hold for a few seconds *(Figure 5)*.

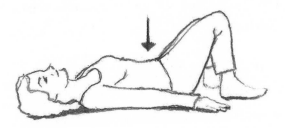

Figure 5

Bridging

When I don't have hip nerve pain, I also bridge several times, immediately after pressing my low back to the floor and pulling in my abdomen. Bridging is a very good way to strengthen the core muscles, which will take some of the pressure off the back and also assist a limp. It's a bit difficult if your core muscles are weak, but over time we all get better at it. It's best not to do this while having a sciatica episode, but when you are feeling okay, this can actually help to prevent sciatica and low back pain. The stronger our core is, the easier standing or walking becomes. Harvard Women's Health has a good booklet on core strength and power training exercises; in fact, they have several great health-related publications. (See Bibliography.)

To bridge: Lie on the floor, arms at sides, bend your knees, and pull your feet a few inches toward your hips. With your feet flat on the floor and shins essentially perpendicular to the floor, pull your belly button area toward your backbone and hold firmly, breathe out, and lift your pelvis with shoulders still flat on the floor. Your arms will serve as further support in keeping your hips off the ground *(Figure 6)*. Hold for several seconds, then slowly lower your hips.

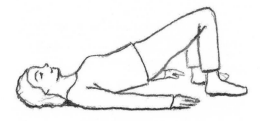

Figure 6

When holding the bridge pose, imagine a line that starts just below your shoulders and goes straight through your body up your thighs to your knees. Your back should be straight, with the plane of your chest and stomach forming a more or less straight line and your hips not sagging down toward the floor (which they may do until you are strong enough to make a straight-line bridge). From the side, the space below your torso should look like a long triangle.

I do this bridging pose about five or more times a day, holding for a few seconds. When I first started, I was holding for five seconds and trying to do ten repetitions but found that my weak hip started hurting. (I have a deformed pelvis and hip, and my hips also have some arthritis.) My polio doc also says that for people like me—polio survivors, MS patients, and fibromyalgia and chronic fatigue folks—longer holds rather than more repetitions give better strengthening results. In this way, we are less likely to fatigue. This is essentially what's called isometric exercising—strengthening by contracting muscles intensely and holding, rather than doing many repetitions. So that's what I do now: fewer reps, longer holds. If you're already fairly strong, though, you can do more repetitions plus long holds for greater effect.

If you are doing bridging correctly and effectively, you may get some soreness in your abdomen at first, which means those muscles really need strengthening. If your tummy is really sore, back off and do less. A little soreness is normal, and just means you're workin' it—but strength, not pain, is the point here.

An Active Core Exercise

When lying on your back, put your hands behind your neck, hold your stomach in, and alternately try to touch your right elbow to your left knee (drawing that knee up toward the chest) and then your left elbow to your right knee (*Figure 7*).

Do this quickly—at least five times, but as many as possible without hurting your back. It's not absolutely

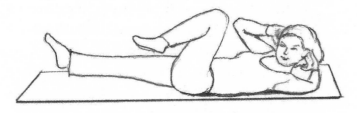

Figure 7

necessary to touch elbow to knee, but if you can, you will get a better workout.

If you feel a tiny bit sore in your abdomen the day after first employing this exercise, you've done enough repetitions. If you don't feel at all sore, do more. If you're having sciatica, wait till it subsides to try this one.

A "Traction" Back Stretch

Still lying on the floor (supine, legs straight), grasp the long edges of a yoga mat, runner rug, or large (beach) towel, letting the horizontal surface position your hips in place while pulling down on the mat toward your toes, causing the back from hips to shoulders to stretch *(Figure 8)*.

You'll see how it works once you try it. It is best done with a rubber mat on a rug or floor so that you don't slide. I do this for about a minute every day.

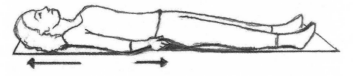

Figure 8

For the Outsides of Your Legs and Hips

For the tendons on the outsides of knees, and also for sciatica nerve pain that runs down the outsides of the thighs, this next position stretches the iliotibial band, the fascia that run all along the top outside of your leg, from hip to below the knee—more commonly known as the IT band.

Lie on your back, raise one leg diagonally and up across your body as far as possible, and hold for at least thirty seconds without twisting your body up off the mat—similar to the first stretch I described, but here positioned with the opposite leg straight on the floor instead of bent (*Figure 9*).

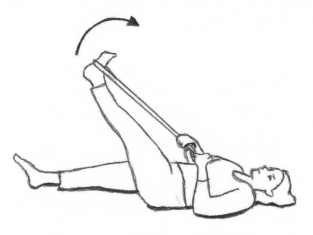

Figure 9

It may be necessary or helpful to take a robe tie, hold an end in each hand, put the middle of the tie under the bottom of your foot, and pull up and over diagonally to get a good stretch. As an alternative to the robe tie, you can either use the opposite hand to pull the foot over or pull your toes up while your leg is crossed over your body; either way, you should feel a stretch along the outside of your leg. After holding for twenty to forty seconds, repeat on the other side. The hip of the raised leg should be the only part of your body raised from the floor (unless you are using a robe tie, in which case your hands and forearms will also be raised).

To stretch the piriformis area (toward the side of the back of the hip, where you sit), lie on your back, cradle your thigh and calf in your arms, and pull your knee up toward your chest and over to the opposite side so that the inside of your ankle is above and perpendicular to your side, or is at least above your abdomen *(Figure 10)*. You should feel a good stretch in the piriformis area. Hold for at least thirty seconds. Then repeat on the other side.

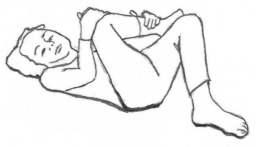

Figure 10

Extra Core Strengthening

Bonus points! I do these extra exercises on the days I'm not going to work out in the pool. I have to be careful not to do too much in one day, since I fatigue easily.

Marching (*Figure 11*): Lie on your back with knees bent, pull in your abdomen (down toward the floor), and lift each knee, alternating between the two, as if you were slowly marching. I only do about eight of these because I have to be careful not to over-fatigue the quadriceps on my weak leg. You can do more if you have strong thighs.

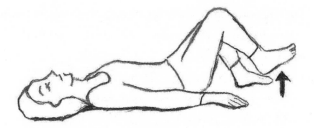

Figure 11

Hip flexion hold and press (*Figure 12*): Next, again hold in your abdomen and then lift one leg so that your calf is perpendicular to the floor and press your palm against your thigh above the knee for a few seconds. Switch to the other leg and do the same. Do a few repetitions.

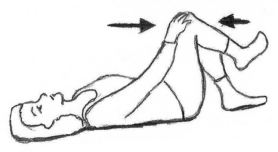

Figure 12

Modified clamshell (Figure 13): The clamshell strengthens the abductor or outer muscles of the hips and thighs. It is normally done lying on your side with legs bent. You then slowly lift the top knee a few inches, or as much as you can, repeating several times. Because my most-affected polio leg is too weak to accomplish this, I do a modified-resistance clamshell.

Lie on your back with legs bent and loop a rubber TheraBand or other stretchy band behind your thighs, below your knees. Hold each end of the band in the opposite hand so the band crosses in front of your thighs, then try to push knees out to the sides while pulling hard on the bands with your hands. Repeat a few or several times.

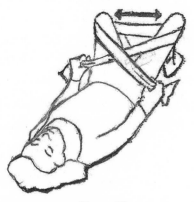

Figure 13

Knees: Some Easy Strengthening

For weak or unstable knees, here are some (more) easy isometrics.

Fold up a hand towel or washcloth, put it under your knee while sitting on the floor, and press the back of the knee down into the towel and hold for a few seconds, at least five or ten, and repeat several times *(Figure 14)*. Repeat on other knee. This helps to strengthen the quadriceps, the muscle above the knee, which helps to keep the knee in its correct position. Knees depend upon the quadriceps for stability.

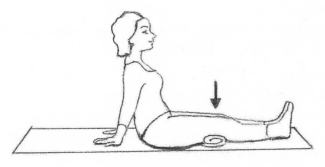

Figure 14

Place a squishy ball (a child's inflated play ball about six inches in diameter) under the knee and press your heel down into the floor for a few seconds, and repeat a few times *(Figure 15; note that the illustration shows the knee higher up than it will actually be with a 6-inch ball)*. This also strengthens your hamstring tendons.

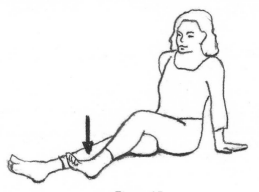

Figure 15

At the end of your knee-exercise portion, squeeze the ball between your knees and hold for ten or more seconds. This strengthens the adductor muscles, the opposite of the ones used in the clamshell exercise. You can do this lying down with knees bent, but I have done it sitting up on the floor with legs straight. A pillow can be used between the knees, though this makes the exercise less effective.

You can also do a ball-between-knees squeeze while sitting in a chair: hold for ten to fifteen seconds, relax, then raise one foot so your leg is out straight and hold again, lower the foot and relax, then raise the other foot and hold. Repeat.

Another great knee exercise is to lie on your back and "write" the alphabet in the air with your foot, keeping your leg straight at about a 45-degree angle. If you can't do the whole alphabet, that's a good sign that your quads are weak, so work up to as many letters as you can, increasing either daily or weekly as much as possible without incurring pain or fatigue. Don't feel bad if you can only get to "F"—just keep at it, daily or weekly adding a few letters.

(Being on the floor in the sitting position is a great time to do foot exercises with a therapy band, as mentioned in Chapter 15.)

Thigh Tendon Stretches

When sitting up on the floor, legs outstretched, lean forward, keeping your back straight, and grip your feet to get a good hamstring (tendons in backs of thighs) stretch, holding for thirty to ninety seconds (*Figure 16*).

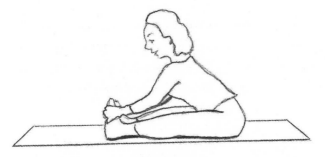

Figure 16

If you can't reach your feet, start by putting your palms on your shins, as low as possible. According to one of my most respected orthopedists, tendons love to be stretched. They are happiest and healthiest (and the least likely to be painful) when we stretch them a bit each day.

After doing the sitting hamstring stretch, spread your feet as far apart as you can, grasp them, and hold for twenty to forty seconds *(Figure 17)*. Again, put your hands on your shins if you cannot reach your feet (yet). I have not been able to get beyond a fifty-degree spread, but I'm still trying. This is a good stretch for inner thighs, also assisting hamstrings to be healthy, because these sets of tendons interact and support each other in not being overworked.

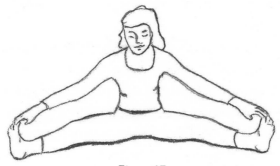

Figure 17

Next, grasp your ankles or feet and pull them toward your body with your heels pointed toward your crotch, soles pressed together, and hold for twenty to forty seconds. This is known as the Cobbler's Pose (*Figure 18*).

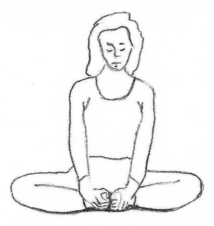

Figure 18

This is also a good time to do Kegel exercises, which help to prevent urinary incontinence (and also, happily, help women to continue to achieve orgasm and men to keep an erection).

More Back Stretching but Prone: Child's Pose

Child's Pose is a good stretch for hips, back, and arms, and also tops of feet. Not everyone can do this pose, and if you don't have the flexibility, either start attempting to stretch into this position a little bit at a time or skip it.

From hands-and-knees position, kneel with feet hip-width apart, tops of feet on the floor. Lean forward and sit down slowly on heels till your head is as close to the floor as possible (forehead on floor if possible, but see second paragraph below for alternatives) with forearms flat on floor and, if possible, buttocks resting on ankles or heels— folded up, essentially (*Figure 19*).

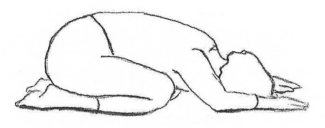

Figure 19

If you can just be on your hands and knees and even start lowering your buttocks down and hold that position for a few seconds, it will be a beneficial stretch. When I first started doing this a decade ago, it was difficult, but after a year or two of daily practice, it no longer was.

With your face on the floor—or as close to the floor as possible—gradually extend your arms as far forward as you can (in front of your head, palms on the floor and elbows off the floor with arms straight; forehead may be lifted off the floor slightly)—this is the Extended Child's Pose (*Figure 20*). I start with elbows at my sides and hold for a few seconds, moving my hands up the mat a little at a time and holding a few seconds at each further stretch. When you get your hands as far forward as possible, hold for as long as you can without pain.

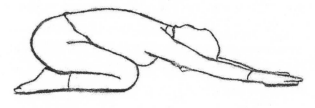

Figure 20

When I first started practicing Child's Pose, I could not get my head to the floor, so I used a pillow, a folded towel, or my two fists, end to end, to support my forehead. It's fine to do it this way! My knees also could not take this position for more than half a minute, so I only held the pose for about twenty-five seconds. I can now stay in Extended Child comfortably for a couple of minutes, with forehead on or near the floor.

Be sure to stop if you experience pain, especially if it is sharp! You should just feel a really good stretch all along your back, hips, tops of feet, sides, and arms.

After holding Child's Pose for as long as feels comfortable, lie down prone (face down) and rest for about 20 percent of the time you've done the pose. I like to put my hands near my face, palms down, with my forearms resting on the floor and even with my forehead resting on the backs of my fingers. I found by experimenting that this 20 percent interim was how long my body needed to recover before the next (difficult) pose.

Planking

This is not easy but is very much worth it for anyone who wants to build the core. The only parts touching the floor when you're doing this exercise correctly are the bottoms of your toes, the backs of your forearms, and the outside edges of your hands (little-finger side). Your legs, back, and torso are held rigid and straight *(Figure 21)*.

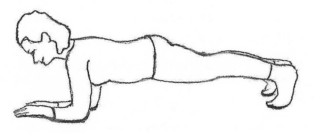

Figure 21

For my own adaptation, I usually rest my polio toes on top of those of my strong foot (as opposed to placing my feet separately), since my little foot has no strength at all.

At first, I could only plank for five seconds; after several months of practice, however, I was up to thirty. If I hold longer, I experience pain in my strong foot's toes, so I sometimes do two planks of thirty seconds each. (Due to shoulder surgery, I had to stop this for a while, but now, after several months, starting with only five seconds, I am back to one plank of twenty to thirty seconds.)

People with two strong feet and arms can usually work up to planking for four minutes or more. I'll never be able to do this; don't feel bad if you can't, either. I tried planking with the tops of my feet on the floor, soles facing the ceiling, toes outstretched, which is supposed to be easier and still strengthen the core—but for me it was nearly impossible, and more painful. A common yoga plank is also done with hands flat on floor so that the arms are straight (perpendicular to floor) and torso is high off the floor.

Cat and Tabletop (Modified Cow)

After Child's Pose or planking, I alternate Cat and Tabletop or Cow poses, on hands and knees, holding each pose just four or five seconds and repeating up to ten times (*Figures 22 and 23*).

Cat has back arched up, stomach pulled in and chin down.

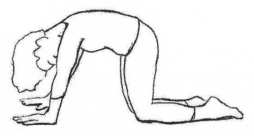

Figure 22

Tabletop or Cow has face looking forward and back straight but stretched long.

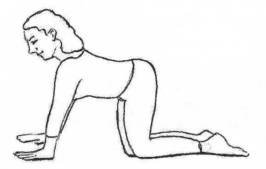

Figure 23

Don't bow or sway your tummy and back down toward the floor when you do Tabletop/Cow, as you may see in some illustrations. Make your back straight and elongated like a tabletop, as in the illustration here. If you have back trouble, it's generally not good to concave arch (hyperextend) your belly or waist toward the floor with hips and head up, which compresses the vertebrae. Arching with your back up and tummy pulled toward your back, in contrast, is generally good and strengthening for your back and, as in some other poses, temporarily makes a little relieving space between your vertebrae.

Icing and Ice Packs

This is my most reliable quick fix for any bodily pain—especially back pain, but also pain in the shoulders or the tendon problem in my strong foot; it's especially good for sprains or breaks, or any injury with swelling. Cold compresses reduce inflammation, thus pain, and make it easier for the body to heal. (If arthritis is the primary problem, on the other hand, that tends to respond better to a heating pad.) I recommend the high-quality, heavy vinyl, black gel ice packs you can find at physical therapy offices and online. The blue ones sold at drugstores, medical supply stores, and also online tend to split open quickly—within two years—at the seams, and the gel leaks out. What a mess. They can be taped with plastic packaging tape, but it's not a great fix and doesn't last. It's much more cost efficient to buy the black ones in the first place. I keep gel packs in the freezer always, as they take two hours to get cold enough to be of benefit.

After placing a thin piece of cotton cloth, such as an old dish towel, between your skin and the ice pack—or while wearing a thin T-shirt—relax, preferably lying down, with the ice or gel pack on the sore area for twelve to thirty minutes. Twenty minutes is usually sufficient, while less than twelve will do little or no good; you really need to get to a state of near numbness in order for the tissues to gain benefit. At first there is sometimes a burning sensation, but if you ride it out, the area becomes numb and even pain-free.

If the pain is acute, ice again after about an hour or two. (This is why you need to have more than one ice pack.) Post-surgery, I have been advised to apply every hour, for a half hour on and a half hour off, for seven to ten days, for which I needed a circulating ice water machine. For injuries such as sprains and breaks, I have been told—and have read, too—that the first forty-eight hours is most crucial, and it's not necessary to ice after that. But in cases where there has still been pain or swelling after that initial period, I have continued to find relief from icing.

Gel-pack instructions say not to lie on top of the pack, but I find that the pressure of my body pushes me into the cold and is most effective. Some physical therapists have had me lie on my stomach, face turned to one side, with the gel pack on my back; I find that this sometimes strains my neck unless I'm lying on a table with a "nose hole" in it, like a chiropractic table, and even then that position is not particularly comfortable.

Ice in one of those old-fashioned ice bags is good, but not very comfy to lie upon; that's better for a knee or other topside body part. You can try multiple layered plastic bags with crushed ice, but I have found that they always leak, no matter what you do. Frozen peas also work, but I'd dedicate a bag for this, since re-freezing foods deteriorates their quality. (Also, peas thaw rather quickly.)

I do have a mini ice bag I purchased online that I use for travel. You can take a small gel ice pack in your checked baggage when you fly, but you can't take bigger gel packs in your carry-on unless you have a written prescription—and even then, you'll be pulled aside for questioning. (They're also quite heavy—not worth the extra hassle.) But you can take an empty mini ice bag in a carry-on, and even get ice from a vendor once you're through security at the airport, and then use it on the plane or while you wait to embark. If you do that, be sure to put the mini ice pack in a plastic bag, because it's likely to leak.

When I've been on my feet too much in a day, arthritis and canal stenosis (narrowing of the spinal canal, which causes a slightly pinched nerve) in my low back can be so painful that I can barely walk. Icing my low back and hip areas often restores them to a natural, non-inflamed, pain-free—or at least reduced-pain—state. I sometimes have to ice my back twice in an evening, but most of the time one session fixes me right up. For arthritis, a heating pad (especially one with moist heat) is usually more effective, but because the nerve pain caused by my canal stenosis is more debilitating than my arthritic disc issue, I find that it's not that helpful for my particular back problems. If you're not sure of the cause of your own back pain, talk to your doctor and perhaps try both ice and heat to see which gives lasting relief. Alternating ice and heat will also improve circulation by causing a "pumping action" in the blood vessels, which facilitates healing as well.

Oscillating Platforms

An oscillating platform may be helpful if you are tending toward osteoporosis or osteopenia in your back, legs, or hips. I use one of these on many of the days I don't work out in the pool. British studies have proven that this device improves bone density. Mine is a SoloFlex, and cost $250 on sale in 2012. I set it at the lowest setting, stand on it for ten minutes, sometimes a few more—that's about as long as I can stand in one place, so that's my realistic time limit—and read a book while I vibrate. (You could also watch TV or listen to music.)

The platform on my device is about four feet long, a foot wide, and four or five inches high, so it easily slips under a long, low dresser or a bed. For bone strengthening, set it on the lowest setting. It gives your body an all-over workout, and you may be surprised to feel a little tired after using it; I generally rest for a couple of minutes afterward.

Easy does it with this equipment; a higher setting may throw you right off the platform, and for bone strengthening it is not additionally beneficial to set it any higher than the lowest setting. Between using this platform and jumping up and down in the pool, where the water absorbs some of the impact and is safer for bones than the jolting impact of jumping on the ground or cement, I have improved my bone-density score. At one point, I even moved from osteoporosis to osteopenia (essentially a midpoint between healthy bones and osteoporosis; bones are getting weaker and less dense but have not reached the deteriorated condition of osteoporosis, when bones become more "porous" and less dense). Bones break easily when their density has become reduced to the state of osteoporosis, so learning that I had improved the density of my own so significantly was pretty exciting. (Cheap thrills!)

Losing Weight

According to several sources—including some of my physical therapists, *Arthritis Today*, and *Harvard Women's Health Watch*—for every pound you lose, you take four or more pounds of pressure off your back and legs, especially your knees, hips, and vertebrae. With that in mind, you're at your best by keeping your body mass index (BMI) below 29 (as long as you keep it *above* 18, which is considered to be "underweight"; this is especially true for seniors, since we need a little extra weight that can be lost in case of illness).

BMI chart:
Underweight = 18.5 or less
Normal = 18.5 to 24.9
Overweight = 25–29.9
Obesity = 30 or more

To calculate your BMI: Multiply your height in inches by height in inches (square of height in inches). Then divide your weight in pounds by square of height in inches, and multiply by 703.

Thus, if you are five feet three inches tall and weigh 150 pounds, 150 ÷ 3,969 x 703 = 26.57, or (rounding up) 26.6. According to the official BMI chart, this puts you at just a bit overweight; ten pounds less would put you in the "normal" range. (Yes, these terms are somewhat charged and not exactly PC—sorry for that. This is not intended to be weight shaming, but an encouragement for being in the best health possible; I do feel the science behind this calculation is sound.) And although that computation was not mine, yes, by these standards, I'm overweight. In fact, I'd need to lose at least 10 percent of my current body weight to put myself in the "normal" BMI category. Unfortunately, this is something that we all face, especially as we grow older and almost always shorter, and it means we have to reduce caloric intake in addition to exercising regularly. Especially unfair for someone who loves buttered popcorn as much as I do. (At least popcorn is better than potato or corn chips, though!)

How to Lose Weight if You Cannot Exercise Much

Generally, if you cut out "white foods" (other than dairy products) when they have been a regular part of your diet, you will drop pounds, even if you do nothing else to lose weight. (People who eat a lot of dairy find that they also lose weight when they reduce or eliminate these products, but I am not focusing on protein foods here as a weight-gain culprit.) The whites I'm referring to here include all the simple carbohydrates: bread, pasta, potatoes, cookies, cake, foods containing flour, and any form of sugar (including honey, unless we're talking about maybe a half-teaspoon a day). Of all these foods, potatoes actually have some food value, particularly calcium, vitamin C, and potassium, but it's still a good idea to avoid white potatoes if you are overweight. (A couple of small red new potatoes can be added after you lose most of the extra weight.) In the first stages of a weight-loss diet, it's necessary to eat almost entirely lean protein and vegetables, minus the starchy corn and potatoes. As you start to lose pounds, add back whole grains such as oatmeal, brown rice, or whichever whole grains you are able to eat.

Ideally, lean protein or beans, brown rice, quinoa, or other whole grains, coupled with a *lot* of vegetables, should make up the bulk of your regular diet. An Australian study found that people who added about four cups of vegetables and fruits to their diets daily became as happy with their lives as unemployed people who had found a job! So not only is more produce likely to improve your physical health, it also has the potential to improve your state of mind.

Despite this, I would limit fruit till you get to your ideal weight or close to it; fruit has a lot of natural sugar, which you really don't need if you are overweight. Berries are the healthiest and have lowest glycemic levels; apples are not bad, either. Watermelon, bananas, and most tropical fruits have the highest glycemic index, but bananas are a pretty healthy fruit otherwise, so once you start losing, half of a banana now and then is fine. According to the latest information I've read, the only fats that are really bad for you are trans fats, but fat does have a lot of calories. I use olive oil as the main fat in our household.

Some people don't like strong-flavored veggies, such as cruciferous ones (broccoli, cabbage, cauliflower, brussels sprouts); this may be a genetic predisposition which a few people have. Yes, you can now use this as an excuse not to eat them—at least until you read the rest of this paragraph! These excellent vegetables offer great health benefits, so try reducing that bitter taste you dislike so much by roasting them, which will sweeten the taste, or by sautéing them in olive oil and seasonings.

Drink water instead of soft drinks, even the artificially sweetened ones. It's been found that sugar substitutes tell the brain, "You are about to have calories," which leads you to eat more than you would have, because your brain thinks you are hungry and can tell you haven't gotten any calories yet. Same thing goes for using sugar substitutes in your coffee or tea, or in any other foods. Plus, soft drinks deplete your calcium and are also bad for your teeth, which become more precious as we age.

The Mediterranean diet has been proven to be the healthiest. It includes olive oil, fish, a small amount of meat (poultry is best), vegetables, nuts, whole grains, and a little fruit. I actually love to eat this way . . . as long as I don't have to eat much hummus and lemon, and I can have occasional popcorn! Sixteen years ago, I lost nineteen pounds on this diet, so I know it can be done with minimal stress and sacrifice.

As a post-polio patient, I need a high-protein diet; because some of our muscles work harder to make up for the weaker or paralyzed ones, polio patients experience a higher level of muscle stress than the average person, so we need protein as much as athletes do. I do eat limited amounts of high fat and red meats on occasion, but—despite the controversy on saturated fats, which have been recently partially vindicated—I just don't need the calories, given my limitations on exercise (I can't go for walks or ride a bike). So I cook chicken and various types of fish most nights, and we have a small amount of red meat (including pork) about once every ten days.

I have an old cookbook I love called *365 Ways to Cook Chicken*, by Cheryl Sedaker. When I use it, I just update the ingredients with fresher, healthier ones, and avoid the recipes that have ingredients like canned mushroom soup. Another fairly good cookbook is *The 15 Minute Gourmet: Chicken*, by Paulette Mitchell. For fish, although I have at least three fish cookbooks, *The Lady and the Lingcod* by Beverly Seltzer, a fisherwoman in the San Francisco area, is my go-to; it may be out of print, but if you can find one, it's golden. I also clip a lot of recipes from magazines, look up recipes online based on ingredients I have on hand, and keep the recipes Richard and I enjoy the most.

We eat a lot of veggies—I think the best cookbook for them is *Vegetables Every Day* by Jack Bishop. My husband was a veggie avoider but now appreciates that they can be prepared in delicious ways. For starters, use olive oil for sautéing, and throw some garlic in there, too, if you can eat it. With those two ingredients plus a little salt and pepper, many vegetables are remarkably delicious.

Yes, losing weight is not easy to do, but as a healthy diet becomes a habit, it will get easier. You will feel better and your body, especially your back, will thank you after you lose even five pounds. If you have ongoing knee, hip, or back pain and are overweight according to the BMI standards I discussed earlier, a healthier diet is a good way to begin reducing that pain. Plus, the pain will almost certainly get worse if you don't act. You don't want to end up unable to move!

I have struggled with my weight constantly in the last two or three decades. It seems the last ten pounds are the hardest to lose. I do find that rewards help; for instance, telling myself that if I lose three pounds, I can have popcorn, or especially that if I lose five, I can get into my favorite jeans again.

I started doing yoga off and on when I was in my twenties, but I didn't really take it on as a daily practice (i.e., I do it no matter what) until I was around sixty. This daily commitment was largely because I began having back pain and didn't want to have surgery. With that fear motivating me, I added in the stretches and core-strengthening physical therapists taught me, and now they're such a part of my daily practice that they feel as essential as brushing my teeth and feeding my cat. But it takes time to change habits, so don't beat yourself up—or your mom, dad, or spouse—if you or they don't fully incorporate yoga, going for walks, other exercise, or a better diet all at once. Just make one change, and then another, and eventually there will be a day when you'll look back and say, "My back feels better!" or "I've lost five pounds!" or "I have more energy today!"

Good luck with all these self-care practices, and remember: good health, potentially less pain, and a more positive outlook are your real rewards.

Like a Duck Takes to Water:
Healing through Pool Therapy

My primary form of exercise, other than my daily half hour of yoga and core strengthening, is pool therapy. This is almost the only form of aerobic activity that is realistic for me, other than standing to cook, doing grocery shopping, gardening (all of which can cause more back pain), and occasionally dancing for a few minutes. In the pool, I can do stretches, arm exercises, and kicks, as well as walk and swim.

My entire program was set up for me by a physical therapist at a warm-water pool, and then reviewed by a polio specialist.

Gearing Up

In the summer, I slather on a ton of sunscreen in various SPFs; I like Neutrogena Dry Touch best (people often ask me for a recommendation, so I'm plugging here). In the winter, I wear multiple water exercise jackets, or being outside would be intolerable. I have found that H2O Wear has the best selection of jackets, but even so, they aren't great. REI may also have some; if you find a great, lightweight one made of either polyester or neoprene (though I find neoprene too restrictive for active movement) from a different company, please write me at my website! If it's below 60 degrees out, I also wear a fleece and neoprene ski mask until I do my laps. (This is especially important if one has rosacea, which I developed later in life.)

I wear water shoes for jumping and sideways walking. I find that for normal pool walking, they are too heavy on my weak leg. I have purchased them from North Face, REI, and Lands' End, but since one of my feet is child-size, I'm fairly restricted in choice. You just have to try them out to see which ones feel the most comfortable and supportive, and are easy to put on and take off.

The Water's Fine

We were fortunate to be able to install a pool at our home, along with water-circulating solar panels to heat it. We also installed a ramp in the pool instead of stairs for easier access. Polio survivors, with our poorer circulation, are not supposed to exercise in water cooler than 86 degrees Fahrenheit. Some indoor public pools, if used for therapy, are heated to at least this temperature, but most are not. If you have no circulation problems, you may be able to tolerate a lower temperature, but I can only stay in a pool with a temperature of less than 86 degrees for a few minutes.

The drawback in going to a public or club pool, even if it is warm enough for you, is that you have to take all your stuff, drive to the venue, schlep in all the gear, and then schlep it back out when you're done. So if you are generally fatigued, this may not be a good option for you. It worked for me to go to a club pool until they moved all the handicapped parking a quarter mile from the pool. Many public, hotel, and club pools do have a special chair to lower people who cannot walk into the water, however—a big plus for a person in a wheelchair.

My Routine

In establishing how long to do a particular exercise or how many repetitions to do, the polio-advised rule of thumb is to try each exercise separately, *not all on the same day*, and do as many as possible without incurring pain or significant fatigue. Then start the regimen with only 20 percent of that maximum. As that becomes easy, add time or repetitions only a little at a time.

When I started doing this program in 1999, I was able to do about two hours per week. I eventually worked up to about seven hours per week by 2015, but this turned out to be too much; I was becoming over-fatigued. Now I do about two hours a week in the winter and about three to four hours a week during the spring, summer, and fall—sometimes more, if I'm feeling strong enough.

For illustrations of these and other pool exercises, please see either or both of the following books, available on Amazon: *Aquarobics,* by Glenda Baum and W. B. Saunders, or *The Water Workout Recovery Program,* by Robert

G. Watkins, MD, Bill Buhler, and Patricia Loverock. They are chock full of excellent, clear illustrations for those of you with a pool or access to one. (See my Bibliography.)

Here's my program, which is all based on the 20-percent-of-maximum calculation I described above. Times are given for the shortest to longest sets I do. I don't bother getting in the pool if I don't have at least twenty-five minutes to spend in there, and the longest set I can do without exhausting myself is a little less than ninety minutes.

> **1. I begin by walking back and forth in the shallow end for three to eleven minutes.** Sometimes I walk briskly and sometimes slowly, alternating speeds for more aerobic effect. Ideally this should be in waist-high water, but I'm short, so it actually comes up to my rib cage in our pool. (A thirty-two-foot pool has to be three and a half feet deep in the shallow end in order to have the deep end's depth be six feet for diving. If we'd had more room, we would have put in a longer pool with a shallower shallow end.) I walk forward for 60 percent of the time and backward for the other 40 percent, or combine back and forth to come up to that proportion. It is easier to walk forward than backward, so it worked out that to meet the 20 percent rule I have to slightly limit the backward walking segment. I do a little skip so that I land a little harder on my polio leg, because that helps to make the bone denser.

2. Next, I stand near the side of the pool in the shallow end and lift one leg straight out in front of me as high as I can, pulling toes up toward me (on my strong foot only—I have no ankle motion on the polio-weakened foot), holding for thirty seconds. This is helpful for the hamstrings. (I hold all stretches throughout my set for about thirty seconds. My original PT told me to do them for a minimum of ten seconds each, but I find that longer is more effective, and more than one discipline I've read about advises older people not to stretch for much longer than thirty seconds.) Then the other leg, same stretch.

The next stretch is done by bending the knee, grabbing the ankle behind the hip with the hand of the same side, and pulling the foot/ankle up as close to the buttocks as possible and holding. A good pull should be felt in the groin and front of thigh (quadriceps). Repeat on the other side.

3. The following three exercises may seem to be for the arms but are equally (or more) for core strengthening. I use a couple of plastic water paddles that have "pinwheels" on each end so that the resistance can be adjusted. Mine are Nordesco Aquaflex, if you want to look them up online to see what I am talking about and/or buy them:

- Stand with feet planted firmly at hip width, knees slightly bent, one paddle gripped in each hand, palms down. Pull the paddles down through the water with palms down and then back up with palms up, with both arms going up and down at the same time. Keep your body facing forward; do not turn to the side at all. Continue for one to three minutes.

- Hold the paddles in front of you with arms bent and elbows at sides, moving them side to side with both hands at the same time, so that the broad part of the paddle is pushing against the water. Continue for twenty to ninety seconds. This is especially good for improving balance and is referred to as "windshield wipers," although the action is more like clearing a table.

- Alternate the paddles with one palm up and one palm down, pulling down with palm down and pushing up with palm up, while doing the opposite on the other side, so that as one paddle comes down, the other is coming up. Continue for anywhere from twenty-five seconds to two and a half minutes.

All of these paddle exercises help to strengthen the core; the paddle action can pull you off balance unless you stand firm in the water, and attempting to do that engages your core muscles.

4. Two more leg stretches:

- Bring one knee up to chest—as in Figure 1 in the yoga section, except standing—and hold for thirty seconds. You can use one arm to hold on to the side of the pool, if you need help balancing. Repeat with the other leg.

- Bring a knee up with calf across your midriff, holding the calf and knee with one or both arms and hands—as in Figure 10 in the yoga section, except standing—and hold for thirty seconds. Repeat with the other leg.

5. I like to do a calf stretch that can either be done with one foot up on a step or on a ramp, if the pool you use has a ramp. I lean forward until I can feel the back of my calf on the straight leg behind me being stretched (with heel pressed down) and hold for thirty seconds. Repeat on the other side, if neither of your legs are paralyzed. I don't do a calf stretch on my mostly paralyzed leg. That one's musculature is already pretty loose, and I already do a hamstring stretch for it in my morning yoga. The strong leg really needs more stretching.

If you have a fallen arch, it's good to stick a small, foam, adhesive-backed arch support (I got mine on Amazon) in your water shoe when it's dry; the support plus the calf stretch will help to reeducate your foot to have a slightly higher, stronger arch.

6. Now I do some squats. I find that it's best to stand in water that is less than waist-high, so you'll probably need to do this on a step. I do it on our pool ramp, with my shorter leg on the slightly higher side of the ramp, although having my feet on a slanted plane is not ideal.

Hold your arms straight out in front of you, palms down, and squat as low as you can with your butt sticking out behind you, keeping your back straight. It is stressful on your body to keep your back perpendicular to the ground, so angle it at about 30 to 40 degrees. Stand up, then squat again, keeping arms out straight the whole time. Do squat repetitions for fifteen to sixty seconds.

7. In the next exercise, hold on to the side of the pool in the shallow end (we installed some stainless-steel bars, but you can hold on to the coping) and perform these isometric exercises aimed at the buttocks and top backs of thighs—which, incidentally, assist in preventing and relieving tendinitis or tendinosis in those areas.

- Bend one knee and bring that leg's foot up behind you (not holding with your hand this time) so that you can feel an isometric tension at the top back of your thigh/bottom of buttocks, and hold the buttock on that side tight for a few seconds—around twelve does the trick for me. This will only be helpful if you really contract those muscles.

- Now bring the foot back down and raise the leg, keeping it straight, out to the back and slightly to the side, at about a 20- to 30-degree angle, and hold, tightening that buttock.

- The last of these is a little contorted: Put that same leg and foot at a diagonal angle across the back of the other leg as far as you can, with the hip of the leg that's crossed behind dropped down a bit into the water and the foot several inches off the bottom of the pool. Look to the side where the crossed-over foot is pointed, and hold. Then switch to the other leg and do all three isometrics. I do between three and twelve repetitions of all three isometrics, doing about two-thirds of them on my strong side to avoid overworking my weak leg.

8. *Walk sideways in the shallow end, back and forth, for about ninety seconds to five-and-a-half minutes.* It's a good idea to wear water shoes for stability when doing this. As you move your leading foot out to the side, put your toe down first and then your heel, kind of like you might see in a Native American dance. (I am not entirely certain why it's important to do this, but a trusted PT told me to always place my feet this way.)

9. *Hold on to the bars in your pool* (or the side of the pool, if you don't have bars), preferably in the shallow end, with one hand. Slowly and deliberately kick the opposite leg straight up in front of you as high as you can, then bring it back down and kick it out to the side, slowly, as high as you can. Your back should be straight for this; don't lean

forward as you move. Only your leg should move. Continue for fifteen to seventy seconds, and then turn around and repeat on the other side.

10. *Another kick: This one you do with one foot/leg straight out behind you* at about a 20- to 30-degree angle, this time moving your head and torso slightly forward as you kick back but still keeping your back straight. Continue for ten to sixty seconds and then repeat on the other leg.

11. *Move about halfway to the deep end at this point, for more arm work.* The water level ideally should be just below your shoulders. Place a hand on the outside of the opposite arm's elbow, pull the elbow across your body, and hold for about thirty seconds. Repeat on the other side. Then scrunch your shoulders up as high as possible toward your ears and hold for thirty seconds.

12. *Shoulder rolls: Roll shoulders up and around in forward circles* for thirty seconds to two minutes, then roll backward for forty seconds to three minutes. On the last roll, hold your shoulder blades (scapulae) so they're pinched together, with shoulders also down as much as possible, for thirty seconds. A body worker I trust implicitly says not to think of pinching your shoulder blades together at the top but more at the middle of your back, at the bottom of the scapulae.

I used to do the forward rolls longer, because in the "maximum calculation" I could do these more than the backward roll without fatigue. But after shoulder surgery, it became clear that it was more useful to do as much backward rolling as possible, which is usually true for most of us who do not necessarily sit up straight every minute of the day. We often need to straighten our backs and hold shoulders down and back, so I have taken up doing this as much as possible, pool or not.

13. *After holding your shoulders back and down, attempt to bring one hand as far as you can up your back,* palm facing out, and the other hand down the back, palm down toward back, with the two hands reaching for each other. Hold, and then repeat in the opposite direction. Before my shoulder injury, I could grab my fingertips in both directions; today, I am in the process of getting this ability back. This is one stretch that is a determinant in elder assessment for independence and being able to dress oneself without help, so even if you never get in a pool, you may want to start attempting to do this daily. It is also a yoga position.

14. *After I noticed weakness in my knees, my polio doctor suggested that I sit in the pool* (on a step or ramp) and raise and lower my feet slowly from the knee, repeatedly, to strengthen my quadriceps. To save a little time, I usually do this at the same time as I do the three shoulder-stretch holds in 13; double exercises for ninety seconds. But they can be done separately if that's too much to concentrate upon at once.

15. Repeat the calf stretch from Step 5.

16. I take my water shoes off at this point, because I'm going to the deep end and I find them a little heavy for this segment. Take a pool "noodle," those four- to five-foot-long, three-inch-in-diameter, colorful, firm, cylindrical foam things you see kids use and which are also often used in water exercise classes. You can get larger diameter ones, and you may feel safer floating on those if you are not a strong swimmer, but I like the smaller ones because they are more comfortable under my arms.

With the noodle across your front and bent under each armpit, "march" in the pool, bringing up one knee and then the other, for about forty seconds to two and a half minutes. This is a good time to alternate doing fast and slow, to get a more aerobic workout (recently touted as "bursting" and said to be great for circulation and the heart). When you're done, take a break for a few seconds if you've done a longer set of marching, and hang there—it can also be very relieving to a painful back to hang on the noodle in the deep end.

17. "Bicycle" for twenty-five to ninety seconds, also doing bursts of speed.

18. Do a scissor kick, but with both legs out to the sides at the same time, raising your feet as high as you can in the water—kind of like a jumping jack. Kick for twenty to eighty seconds.

19. Now move on to a real, forward-and-backward scissor kick, one leg to the front and one to the back, which some water exercise classes refer to as a "cross-country ski" movement. Do this for fifteen to sixty seconds.

20. Last deep end kick: Get to a corner and put your arms up along the two sides of the coping, with legs down along the pool walls. Holding your abdomen in, lift one leg slowly, bending at the hip, as you did for the shallow-end leg raise, but don't hold it—bring it right back down and then bring the other one up. Do this for about ten to forty-five seconds. This exercise strengthens the stomach muscles when done correctly.

21. Time for laps. I wear a cap and goggles; I've found that the best ones for me are made by Barracuda. The foam-lined goggles don't leave lines on your face, are efficient for keeping water out once you get the strap adjusted and tightened appropriately for your face and head, and you can also adjust the distance between each eye's goggle. Since I'm small-featured, this makes a big difference for me. I buy silicon earplugs (with wings; they keep out the water but still allow me to hear somewhat) from Barracuda as well; they're the best I've found on the market. I also like their rubber caps; I don't care for silicon caps, though I know that many people do.

I have six different swim strokes: American crawl or freestyle, breaststroke, sidestroke, backstroke (not the full pinwheel type, but the one where you bring your arm back straight over your head and then bend at the elbow with a sharp, downward movement through the water to propel the body), frog on the back (easiest of all), and, my favorite, the butterfly. That's the one that really gives your body a good workout, but if you can't do it, skip it. After nearly two years of shoulder injury, surgery, and rehab, I am nearly ecstatic to find that I can finally accomplish it again.

Swimming, when done with correct form, is great arm and all-over aerobic exercise. It is also easier on the joints than impact aerobics such as running and gym aerobics classes.

I swim for two to eleven minutes. When I'm getting out, I do another calf stretch. And that's it!

After a shower, I sometimes recline and rest for a few minutes, and I try to remember to refuel with complex carbohydrates and lean protein as well—if nothing else, a few nuts and a little fruit.

After doing this program for a year or so, I found that I was stronger and less fatigued. Water exercise is also essential in helping me keep my weight down (although, like most people, I have to also limit my calorie intake to actually lose weight!).

Mike and Me

Here's an audacious and incongruous comparison—five things I, the partially paralyzed polio survivor, have in common with Michael Phelps, the Olympic swimming champ:

1. *We have the same arm-span-to-height ratio:* the length of our outstretched arms, measured to our middle fingertips, is greater than our height—though his difference is about six inches and mine is less, naturally. This "monkey arm" ratio is unusual, and useful for powerful swimming. In my case, the reason this probably happened is that I was meant to be two inches taller. If my right leg had not been stunted by polio, I would likely have grown to that height.

2. *Our favorite stroke is the butterfly* ('cause, long arms). I love to watch Phelps's signature propulsion dolphin kick, which I can't quite do but sometimes modify my kick to imitate.

3. *We count strokes, which is useful when your goggles get water in them* or whenever you cannot see

the end of the pool; you can also use counting to keep from hitting your head when on your back. (Counting is almost imperative if you want to be competitive—which I don't.)

4. When we're not swimming as a practice, we don't enjoy going in oceans, rivers, lakes, or other pools "for fun," because we already spend so much time in water; working out (and being wet for a couple of hours a day) is fun enough.

5. We have both smoked pot (me in the past, him, maybe not just the past; no judgment here).

That's it—but given that you'd think we'd have little in common at all, it's a lot, isn't it?

❧

It's fortunate that I love to swim, but even those who are not swimmers or who are afraid of getting in the deep end can walk and do stretches in the water. I am fortunate to have a warm-water pool right in my backyard, and was also lucky to have neighbors who generously let me use their pool at any time when I was a teenager. However, for decades prior to my current living situation, I found that I was always able to locate a publicly accessible warm-water pool in which to do my routine. Although schlepping the gear can be a bit of a drawback, a lightweight rolling duffel bag works really well for this purpose, and will fit in most gym lockers. So do a little research, find yourself a good pool, and dive in.

Okay, you don't have to *dive* in. But do get in and get wet. I promise you'll feel better right away—and probably meet some other nice water birds, too.

Different-Sized Feet,
and Bracing

———○○○○○———

*M*y feet are approximately four sizes apart. I wear a size 6½ in women's on my strong, less-affected foot, which translates to a 5 in youth sizes, and I wear a 2 in women's or youth's on the other foot. This means that my only options for buying matching shoes are to buy two pairs in the youth-size range, or have shoes made.

I researched having a pair of flats made by a medical orthopedic organization in San Francisco a few years ago; the cost was $1,200 to $1,500 a pair . . . for flats. And that was around 2015; I can only imagine that the cost has gone up. It has been my intention to see if another shoemaker would make them for a lesser price, but the only times I've had boots made for me—once in the 1970s and once in the '90s, by shoemakers here in the SF Bay Area—they caused me foot pain or the heels were too high to be safe.

Although it is extremely difficult for me to get matching shoes that are comfortable for each of these two very different feet (it's like buying a pair for your grandmother and your eleven-year-old daughter—who has a paralyzed foot—all at once), I do occasionally buy two pairs.

If you or your favorite Wild Handicapper has a similar problem, even if the feet are only a half-size different, you might find the following information helpful!

Buying Shoes for Mismatched Feet

The only place I know of where you can buy shoes in two different sizes and only pay for one pair is Nordstrom. If you find an identical pair in your two different sizes, they will split the pair and send back to the manufacturer the mis-mates you can't use. You pay for the more expensive pair, but it's a much better deal than paying double! If you use Nordstrom online, you buy the two pair first and then include a letter when you ship the mis-mates back to Nordstrom, telling them that you are wearing one shoe from each pair, and they credit you for the cost of the cheaper pair. I find that this often confuses them, resulting in their crediting me for two pair instead of one, since they have received two boxes, even though each box has only one shoe in it; I contact them if they make the mistake, and if they don't re-charge me, it's their problem at that point.

The other best place I have found to shop for shoes, maybe even better in some respects, is Zappo's. If you order more than $50 worth, which of course you will if you order at least two pair, shipping is free. They provide free return shipping labels online. You cannot split up the pairs, but at least you can try out a lot of shoes without going to several stores and using your precious energy. All you have to do is to box your returns and drop them off at a UPS center, or have someone do that for you.

I buy nearly all my double-pair shoes from Zappo's or Nordstrom online. I've also had some luck with Merrell for hiking boots, and with Amazon and Lands' End for water exercise shoes, though I've liked REI's water sandals better until recently. For me, it is not worth it to expend the physical energy required for shopping in person, especially with the free returns offered by some online retailers.

I send back 80 percent of what I buy. The extra mismatched shoes that cannot be returned to anyone (except Nordstrom) can be donated at full value for a charitable tax deduction to National Odd Shoe Exchange in Chandler, AZ. You may be able to get shoes from them, too; I have not had good luck in that regard in the last fifty years, though they did pair me up with a mis-mate partner when I was in high school. Worth a try, anyway.

Flats cost me around $60 a pair (so that's $120, when I'm not buying from Nordstrom) unless they're made of better material, in which case they can cost double that. Once I've found the shoes, I pay about $60—which is a very good rate, at least in the Bay Area—to get the right shoe built up to slightly diminish the length difference in my legs. (I cannot get the full difference corrected or I will turn my ankle, and the lift has to be the same amount on every pair of shoes, regardless of height of heel, so I only correct about 25 percent of the difference.)

If you've done the math, you can see that a pair of girls' Mary Janes costs me about $200. I buy two pairs of the limited selection that fit me and send the odd shoes I can't wear to the National Odd Shoe Exchange. Yes, it's a charitable contribution, but I'm still out about 75 percent of the cost of that second pair. It's not ideal, but I've had a lifetime to get used to it.

How to Deal with a Drop Foot

Not only polio survivors but also stroke survivors and sometimes people who have nerve damage due to back surgery often end up with what is known as a "drop foot." This is a foot that cannot be raised up or pressed down; it essentially just hangs there, usually at a less than 45-degree angle to the leg.

In order to get bracing for this, one needs to get a prescription from a doctor to see an orthotist and be fitted for an ankle/foot orthotic (AFO), a lightweight fiberglass or plastic brace. Some are heavier or bigger than others, depending on the wearer's condition, size, and activity level and the types of shoes that will be worn. In some cases, it will be necessary to replace all shoes to wear with this brace. That is what happened for me when I got one in 1988; I had to throw out probably ten or more pairs of shoes that would not have been of use to anyone because of the size differences.

The AFO I wear (which I discussed in greater detail in *Not a Poster Child*) supports the bottom of my foot, but is made of firmer material than an arch support, and also has a wide vertical piece that extends up the back of the leg, with small "wings" around the calf. A Velcro strap attached to the wings completes the circle around the calf, and easily secures the AFO in place. This holds the drop foot in a more normal position, which helps the wearer avoid catching the toe and tripping and alleviates the need to lift the hip to facilitate the toe clearing the floor. Not only does this mean better ankle support, it also means less fatigue on the entire leg. It is important that the orthotic be lightweight enough that it not cause more strain on a weak thigh and hip.

Dynamic Bracing Solutions

This system involves heavy bracing on the legs, somewhat like a modified exoskeleton for people with extreme weakness or partial paralysis in one or both legs. It was originally designed by a physicist and has been taken to the next level by a brace maker in Southern California. A former physical therapist and polio survivor presented both her own experience and a video to my polio group featuring someone who not only walked much better with the braces but whose legs have become stronger as a result of the gait correction. It appears that some people who have stuck with the arduous learning curve gain stamina and strength. The presenter was in her late sixties, and she said that she'd gone from having pain after walking a quarter mile to being able to walk three miles with no pain with the brace. (She had far more ability after her bout with polio than I ever had; she contracted it later in childhood, so there was less damage to growth, and she had a less severe case. But two others using the system came to the meeting and also attested to its power to help people stand and walk.) One drawback about this bracing is that it costs a lot—at least $10,000, and up to $40,000 for a set for both legs. But it has changed lives, and if enough people start requesting it, perhaps eventually it will be at least partially covered by Medicare or other insurance.

I had an evaluation for this system by the brace maker and talked it over with my polio physiatrist. She felt, and I saw in my x-rays, that my hip is too malformed and weakened to be able to take the stress of the brace, which I could feel in the positioning required in the evaluation. This is because at the hip joint, my pelvic ilium and top-of-leg femur bones grew out in an extended and flattened fashion to make up for the length difference in my legs, so I don't have a normal ball-and-socket function at that joint. (Yet another argument for vaccinations.) I was very disappointed not to be a candidate, but the bracing system is simply not for everyone.

Although many people do have a half-size difference between their feet and have lived with stuffing a shoe or having one constantly slip off one foot for years, it's pretty unusual for anyone to have the vast foot-size differences I do. Drop foot is not all that common, either. Still, I know that other drop-footers and different-sized-feet folks are out there, and I'm hoping that some of my suggestions in this chapter will be something you or your Wild Handi-capper finds useful.

PART 3:

Participating in Community

Groupie—Finding Your Flock

———·····oO◯Oo·····———

I 've always been a joiner. It's only in the last two decades that I've realized I primarily get more regeneration from being alone than I do from being in groups of people; for most of my life, I've gravitated toward various groups.

Flock Hopping

First, there were church groups—for little kids, then big kids, then teenagers. I skipped the adult experience. My favorite experience in the children's church group was embroidering a sampler on burlap that read, in three lines, "Greet the day with a song; Make others happy; Serve gladly." That represented the ideal Christian girl—one I very much wanted to be at that time.

I joined Bluebirds in grade school, which may have been my mom's idea, or I may have wanted to join because my friend Daralyn was in Camp Fire Girls, the older girls' version. At eight, I had to join Bluebirds first. Bluebirds was slightly patriotic, mostly social, and artsy-crafty. Then we graduated into Camp Fire Girls, where we earned beads for various accomplishments and service: hospital corners on the sheets (I've taught my housecleaner; she's making an effort but so far, no bead); reading the newspaper every day for a week for citizenship, the red, white, and blue bead; and making a cake on your own for a homemaker's bead, probably an orange one.

Although I enjoyed many aspects of Camp Fire Girls, it was also full of humiliating events for me—such as being reprimanded loudly by our leader in front of the entire group for eating a blanched, salted almond off a tray full of them in readiness for the annual fundraiser Christmas fair. Everyone in the kitchen turned and stared at me, my face went red as a beet, and then we carried on. Perhaps my Camp Fire leader may have been going out of her way to make sure I didn't think I could get away with anything because I was handicapped. She needn't have worried; I knew well that I didn't get a free pass.

Another time, when I was about eleven, the group leader's daughter noticed me picking my nose and suggested I blow my nose before school in the morning, as she did—she of the perfect ponytail and straight teeth. She truly meant to be kind, and told me very quietly when we were alone in the backseat of her mother's white Cadillac, but I was mortified. I did, however, learn not to pick my nose in public.

This is the advice my mom might have been giving me, if she had not been so overwhelmed—with grief, at my father's untimely death, and by keeping our household afloat financially. Looking back, I'm guessing that we (especially my mother) were pitied because she was raising a handicapped child alone and running my dad's business to boot. I began to feel that I fell far below the social standard required for a girls' group. Even so, I deeply loved the camping aspect of Camp Fire Girls, and a few years after I quit the organization as a regular member, I went back as a camp counselor. Nothing like walking in the woods (to the extent I could) and singing around a campfire. I still remember the songs we sang. One in particular, "The Call of the Fire," was most haunting and beautiful. It captured the peace and solitude of the great outdoors and was sung in a minor key—always a hook for me.

I joined choruses at school from fourth through eighth grade, auditioning first at nine and again at twelve. In high school, I was in a folk group rather like the Christy Minstrels and learned basic guitar. That was particularly fun since in our senior year we got to skip school once in a while as ambassadors from the school to sing at women's clubs and for civic groups.

I took a hiatus on groups for some years in my twenties and thirties, in college and after, though I did go to Vietnam protests and also joined a co-op in the early 1970s, where I learned about organic produce and recycling. (To me, not recycling is much worse than not believing in a deity.) I sang in a number of choirs or choruses, both community and smaller—classical, rock 'n' roll, and jazz—in the 1980s and '90s.

And then there were the Sufis, a mystical group that believes we are all one with God, that God actually *is* love, the glue that holds the universe together, and that one of the most important philosophies of life is to learn to see from the point of view of another. This philosophy is an offshoot or subset of Islam, but a westernized and non-orthodox version. It's based on teachings of Muslims who studied in India and incorporated breath work, yoga, and singing and chanting of holy names into their practice. Western Sufis study Christianity, Judaism, Buddhism, and most world religions, and some may concentrate on one of those even more than Islam. It's more about dropping religious concepts and living, feeling, one's belief in unity.

I took initiation in this "way of the heart" in 1976, while attending college and working nearly full time. I was very active for two or three decades and spent four years in the Sufi Choir, which integrated my love of music with spirituality—a fine marriage indeed. Now I mainly participate in a Sufi-oriented women's group (the Luscious Fruitcake Mamas). We meet a few times a year, do some spiritual practices, share what's current in our lives, and have a potluck schmooze. It meets my need for spiritual community.

I joined my current "other" women's group, which has a brother men's group (to which my husband, Richard, belongs), in 1991, and have attended nearly every month since. The purpose of the clubs is to learn to listen with compassion so that we have an experience of being loved by a group. By keeping our opinions or assessments to ourselves as we listen (not easy, but we do our best), we get to consider what our positions are and how they may or may not lead us to greater compassion, and the speaker gets to feel known and more fully understood than she usually might. We don't refer to it as a support group, but it may fit the definition.

It certainly is a deep emotional support for me to be truly known, warts and all, with very little judgment. Being listened to with compassion is remarkably liberating. When people are listening with intent to correct, or to offer advice, or even share their own experience (guilty, here, on that third one), or with disdain, it is felt, and speaking can become frustrating rather than healing. That is not the case in this group. When we do have a consideration about the speaker's wisdom, are concerned for their welfare, or think of a similar experience we've had, we say, "Can I ask you a question [or "make a suggestion" or "make a comment"]?" The speaker sometimes says no, she just wants to be heard; but sometimes she asks for insights. I have found my experience in this group to be perfect and have become more deeply attached to the women who belong to it with each year's passing.

I joined the local chapter of the California Society of Enrolled Agents in 1991 after passing the IRS's enrolled agents' exam, a two-and-a-half-day exam on federal taxation. (This didn't mean we worked for the IRS; it meant we'd been tested on about five times as much taxation as most CPAs and attorneys.) In the Society, we commiserated on tax issues, attended tax seminars, and did a little socializing, but the most supportive aspect of the group for me was a friendly little once-a-month luncheon subset I was invited to join. While we did talk about taxes, and we emailed each other regarding complex tax issues, an especially integral part of the group for me was that we listened to and sympathized with each other when things got rough. Tax season is grueling and should not be attempted alone! I feel fortunate that although I am no longer a tax accountant, they still welcome me at the lunches.

When I had breast cancer, I joined a support group (no surprise). I read in the research I did on the disease that women (and men) in breast cancer support groups had a longer survival rate and withstood the rigors of treatment better than those who "did it all on their own." I soon found in the group that while it was not unusual for someone to cry if they felt the need, there was so much more than sympathy going on. We shared our experiences, recommendations for the best doctors, which tests our doctors had run on our biopsies, and more, which led to some discovering that doctors were not running tests that could be necessary or helpful in designing specified treatments. Getting a second opinion was something everyone who'd had a second opinion recommended.

Learning that there were so many ways to face cancer was enlightening, too: some women in the group studied every single thing they could get their hands on and some just let a doctor or series of doctors tell them what to do, where to go, and when to do it all. The group respected each woman's choices in that regard. We laughed a lot—the black humor of women facing a potentially life-threatening illness.

One of the women in our group had two small children. During chemotherapy, she became more and more tired, and her hands got so blistered from neuropathy that she could not do the dishes, even while wearing gloves. She'd been trying to keep up with everything while going through this debilitating and scary process. She finally had to show her hands to her husband—who was in total denial about the seriousness of her illness—and ask him specifically to do the dishes throughout the rest of her treatment. He was surprised, and grumpy about taking on this task, but he did it. Then he got a bee sting one evening. She shook her head as she told us of how he panicked when his finger swelled and began to throb. "You'd have thought he was going to die," she said—and this was not one of those allergic reactions where he really could have died. There was a moment of silence in the group while we reflected on the gravity of the situation. Then someone said somberly, "Well, but . . . did you get a second opinion?"—followed by our riotous laughter.

These support groups are not pity parties, as some may think. Groups like these are effective because they're places to talk about things that only people with similar experiences can truly understand. The potential solutions one finds in these meetings—whether in how to deal with a relationship difficulty, how to deal with grief, how to deal with personality issues dating back to childhood, how to live with an alcoholic, or how to get your biopsy tissue tested for hormone-receptive cancer growth—can even be lifesaving.

After my own positive experiences of participating in previous support groups, I started two groups myself. I'll tell you how it's done, because I'd like to encourage you to do the same, or to participate in an existing group, whether it's for post-polio, MS, chronic fatigue, genealogy, songwriting, or whatever it is for which you'd like to share support.

Getting Started

I looked for a post-polio support group when I could not find a doctor locally who knew anything about tendon stress and pain in polio patients, specifically in my strong leg and foot. My previous orthopedic surgeon had retired from his practice and all the orthopedists I had found in Marin County looked at my strong leg and suggested that I do things I could not do without a second strong leg.

I found a Northern California post-polio group in the next county up from mine (Sonoma), but they had stopped meeting because so many of them were elderly, tired, and debilitated and most did not have the energy to manage, run, or even attend a group. I went to their swansong luncheon. About forty polio survivors attended, some with their spouses. It was a little strange to be in a room where nearly everyone limped or was in a wheelchair! (It was stranger still, though welcome, when I later attended a polio patients' conference in St. Louis of several hundred.) It was also inspiring to see that many polio survivors live into their nineties and continue to enjoy life, despite having to use a wheelchair or walker. They may have a harder time getting around than other seniors, but they are still getting around! I had not known previously whether simply having had polio was going to mean a shorter life span. What I've learned is that it can for those who need to use ventilators to breathe well, but a shorter life is certainly not the standard. One does have to plan especially well for life as an older person, though. Polio, MS, stroke, chronic fatigue, and similarly conditioned patients need to expect more adaptations and earlier need for assistance.

At that luncheon, I gathered information for folks who lived near me—one of the directors of the Northern California group in Sonoma kindly contacted the Marin County members for me and asked them if she could give me their email addresses or phone numbers. I then emailed the list (and called the few oldest among them whose email addresses had not been provided), telling everyone that I wanted to start a group where we could all share our current condition with each other and possibly pick up some tips as well. I also expressed interest in compiling and sharing a list of medical professionals each member had found to be either knowledgeable about polio or willing to learn about it to help us find creative solutions. It was clear to me that the people who know the few doctors who fit this description would be polio patients themselves. My many calls to local doctors had garnered little.

One challenge when it was time to hold our first meeting was locating a place with no stairs. I also found that most churches charged for use of rooms, but many businesses did not. I originally found a local business that had an elevator and a good-size parking lot with several disabled person parking spots, which we used until that building was sold. I then located an accessible meeting room at a local bank, a contact suggested to me by a disabled persons' support center called the Center for Independent Living (many banks allow non-profit groups to use their conference rooms for free; the Post-Polio Syndrome (PPS) group in Sonoma had non-profit status through another disability group, and I learned that we could call ourselves a non-profit affiliate because we were a satellite of the Sonoma PPS group). We still use this bank conference room, which is at street level and has ample, and close, parking.

To determine a good meeting time, I polled the group and made simple lists and charts using the very scientific "checkmark on most popular days" method. (Polling is the most time-consuming part of starting any group.) I finally discerned days and times that the largest number of people could attend, and we had our first PPS Marin meeting, which eight of the fifteen or so people I'd contacted attended. We all told our stories of when and how we'd contracted polio, briefly shared our current difficulties, and decided to meet once a quarter, attempting to accommodate people's previous commitments.

Later, we compiled the list of medical professionals, which I typed up and emailed to everyone on the list. (New members now receive this, along with a list of members who are willing to share their email addresses and phone numbers, when they join.) I then printed out a set of large postcards and mailed them to several physical therapy, orthotics, and orthopedic offices, with an accompanying note asking them to please let their polio patients, if any, know that we had organized a support group for polio survivors.

I received some inquiries as a result of the card, and between that and word of mouth, our group now has about forty members. Recently, we changed our name from Marin PPS (for Post-Polio Syndrome or Sequelae) to Polio Survivors of Marin, since several people in the group do not have symptoms of post-polio sequelae but are still interested in being included. We learned through Post-Polio Health International, a national organization, that for the most part, polio patients prefer to be called polio survivors rather than "polios," as was common in years past, or even "post-polios."

Although mostly we do not socialize in this group other than engaging in a bit of chat before or after the meeting, or occasional emails between individuals, we do all think of each other and contact one another when a news article or other piece of information is relevant. Some people carpool to the meetings, and some who have things in common other than our shared disability have formed friendships with one another. (I find it annoying when people who are not handicapped think that just because two people are disabled, they should date or would love to be friends. We definitely have many interests that are more important to us than our difficulties, just like normies.)

We do have each other's backs in this group. In one case, a member was having difficulty with Social Security and her health insurance program. We rallied and found resources for her, including free legal advice. Another member suggested to us all a recommendation for a local shoe store that specialized in supportive footwear (if both feet were adult-sized). We also get motivation from one another: it was particularly inspiring, for example, since some of the people in the group are overweight—a hazard of not having full mobility—when one member went on an anti-inflammatory diet, lost nearly a quarter of her weight, and found that her fibromyalgia disappeared along with the extra pounds.

Most of our meetings are attended by six to ten people. We have communication with other polio groups out of the area, and if their meetings have a speaker or other information that is of interest, a member who has attended that group gives a report. I find speakers on topics related to polio, disability, and aging, when possible. I sometimes write up notes when we get such speakers and email them out to the entire group afterward. Some other polio groups also have newsletters, which we share at our meetings or, if they're in email format, forward them to our group. In this way, people do not have to actually attend in person in order to get value from being in the group, which is important since it's difficult for some to attend meetings, whether because of their work schedules or physical limitations. Recently, due to COVID-19, we conducted a Zoom video meeting from our homes. It was successful enough that it may become our norm, since it means those who have difficulty getting to our meetings in person are more likely to attend.

Our local Vivalon (also known as Whistlestop; a seniors' organization) newsletter has been a good source of information, classes, and speakers, and even free or low-cost transportation, as has the Center for Independent Living, a related organization. (Please see Resources for more info on post-polio groups.)

Organizing Online

The other group I started is a group for writers that I organized through Meetup, an online organization with a myriad of get-togethers offered. If you are looking for bird watching, poetry, hiking, concert appreciation, whatever it is, you can probably find it on Meetup. A friend had told me of a particular group where people got together and told each other what they were writing, then wrote for two hours and checked in again at the end. I needed something like this, because I was not finishing my first book; I was only writing when on vacation, which was a pretty sparse commitment!

It turned out the groups my friend had mentioned were just about everywhere *except* Marin County, so I eventually started a Meetup group with this purpose. I used the name Just Write Marin County, and that's what we do: we just write. (Sometimes we also talk a little outside the group, share writing one-on-one, and share publishing and promotion tips and info on writing workshops; some members have made friends in the group.) Being in a group that meets regularly has made me more productive and led me to address my writing goals more realistically. We have also had, from time to time, other Just Write Meetups in Marin, run by other facilitators, that I don't have to maintain.

Although it takes effort to get a group started, once it gets rolling, maintaining one doesn't require much effort. There are always one or two energetic members who will offer to help when needed, too. One of the members of my post-polio group, for instance, set up a Facebook page for us so that other polio survivors might find us (Polio Survivors of Marin—it's brand-new, so at this point few people have "friended" us, but it's a place for us to post about our quarterly meetings as well).

Although, as a somewhat reclusive introvert, my favorite type of hanging out will always be with one to six people, larger groups—particularly support groups—can be a boon. If you have started a group yourself, and no one comes or shows interest, change the name and try again, or broaden the topic. Just give it a go. With a little effort, you too can be a groupie.

Activism and Advocacy

———————◦◦◦◦◦———————

I realized in writing this book that as an activist of sorts for those with disabilities, even one who's only attempting to inform about the issues, it's unrealistic not to address political life at least a little.

I have always been of a somewhat patriotic bent. My father was in the US Navy in World War II, and we watched a lot of anti-Nazi movies when I was in grammar school. Because my parents were Republicans in the 1950s (and, in my mom's case, into the '60s), when that primarily meant "Eisenhower Republican" or fiscally conservative, I thought, as a child, that the GOP was the only party that was right.

But by 1965, after a short right-leaning stint, I was listening to Bob Dylan and Joan Baez, and it was impossible for me not to hear their calls to awareness as the Vietnam War began taking my friends, both into service and into the grave. By the time I started college in 1966,

I was leaning far left. I signed up for an anti-nuclear organization and for Students for a Democratic Society (SDS)—and although I never even attended a rally, I am told my signature probably generated an FBI file on me, since SDS was considered very pinko/commie/socialist. (I just thought it was anti-war and was only beginning to get some idea what socialism might mean at the time.)

I did not like what the United States was doing in other countries; I thought it was imperialist, colonialist, and invasive. And, being very idealistic, I thought that the old men who planned the wars should fight those wars themselves. The Vietnam War did not seem to me as moral as World War II. I wasn't sure if communism had been forced on the Vietnamese, or whether it was a viable system. Today, I'm still not sure if the Vietnamese had a choice, but I'm no longer naive enough to think communism has worked. I do think *some* socialistic policies are workable and intelligent, however.

I didn't really think much about disability rights at that time. I was able to walk with a little more ease then, for one thing. I also thought that physical and social discrimination was something I'd leave in my small hometown with my childhood, and that my new college and adult world would be full of mature, intelligent, unbiased people (and young men who would not care that I was physically defective). I was trying so hard to be like everyone else that my self-image did not include identifying with the group called "disabled."

It would be a couple of decades before I'd sit in a workshop and listen to one person after another share their impressions of my handicap and what it meant to them and emerge stunned by the concepts people had—that because I had a weak, paralyzed leg and was sensitive I must be sad, I must be angry, I must be depressed, I must want people to help me all the time. People who knew me knew that I was, if anything, too independent and unwilling to ask for help. When I finally learned what strangers thought about handicapped people, and that there was a deep prejudice about disability—even among very aware, conscientious people—it was both enlightening and shocking. (Further, I have learned in recent years that some disability rights people stridently do not like to be called "handicapped," which is my preferred term, because I think it indicates ability while needing an allowance for limitation. So even within the disability community, there's dissent, and possible prejudice, around terminology.)

I didn't know in my twenties that Ed Roberts, a polio survivor who is often called the father of the disability rights movement, was nearly denied a high school diploma because he had not completed physical education or drivers' ed (he was in an iron lung). I didn't know that when he applied to UC Berkeley in the early 1960s, he was nearly rejected due to a snide comment—"We've tried cripples before and it didn't work"—from a dean to another administrator.

Roberts was the first severely disabled student to attend UC Berkeley. His iron lung caused him housing difficulties, so he was offered a room in Cowell Hospital—to which he agreed, with the stipulation that his room be treated as a dorm. (Go, Ed!) In 1966, before the free speech movement at UC Berkeley and the same year I graduated from high school, Roberts got his MA in political science.

I had never heard of Camp Jened, a funky summer camp in New York for disabled teenagers run by hippies, before the documentary *Crip Camp* came out in 2020. In that setting, some of these kids had their first experience of social life with people who were all handicapped or disabled in one way or another—affected by cerebral palsy, polio, spina bifida, and an array of difficulties. *Crip Camp*, produced by Barack and Michelle Obama, chronicles these kids' struggles and fortitude. Out of those experiences emerged a core group that migrated to Berkeley, California, and went on to participate with the Center for Independent Living, formed by Ed Roberts to support the immediate needs of disabled people.

Judith Heumann, a wheelchair-bound polio survivor, was a key mover and shaker at Jened. She had initiated disabled rights demonstrations in New York City in 1972, where she had formed Disabled in Action, and later met Ed in Berkeley. She partnered with him on various projects. These ultimately led to the 1977 demonstrations in San Francisco where disabled people actually risked their health, safety, and even lives to spend the night in a federal building, determined to make themselves heard by the Department of Health, Education, and Welfare. They wanted to get particular existing laws regarding building accessibility cemented rather than scrapped, which HEW was about to do because the laws were "too much trouble, too expensive."

At that time, as is the case to some extent today, disabled people were treated as if they were unintelligent and also contributed nothing to society. You probably know that people with, for example, severe speech limitations can obtain college degrees and also high-level employment, but this was uncommon in the late 1970s. Congressman John Burton made HEW listen to Judith and other disabled persons' testimony, and later Judith testified to congress in Washington. Out of this, non-disabled people joined to support this human-rights issue and Washington began to listen, partly due to the sheer numbers of interested, passionate voters who got involved.

While living in the "I'm Not Really Disabled" bubble in the 1960s, I exhausted myself with the long-distance walks and stairs at San Jose State and, later, California College of Arts and Crafts. I worked hard to keep up with everyone else, as I'd been taught to do (many polio kids were admonished not to expect people to give us any breaks, free rides, or special allowances), and kept my mouth shut about it. It wasn't until the end of my freshman year class scheduling at San Jose, when we had to go to each department physically to get our next semester's classes (and I'd actually spent the night on the sidewalk in front of the art department to get my first-year art classes, popular with graduating seniors who needed units), that a wise teacher approached me and quietly said, "You can pre-register; didn't anyone tell you that? You don't have to do all this walking." She didn't say, "Because you are handicapped or disabled," and I appreciated that she didn't draw more attention to me than my limp already did.

There had been nothing in my application that asked if I had a disability, and nothing had been mentioned at freshman orientation about this pre-registration option. I am guessing that college materials now, in this twenty-first century, at least mention accessibility and where to ask the questions one may have as a physically challenged student, but in my young adulthood, no one before that teacher had suggested anything like this to me.

In the mid-1970s, when I was in my late twenties and attending Sonoma State University, I discovered the Disability Resource Center, which was like a Disabled Students' Union. There, the center's cofounder and director, Anthony Tusler, educated me about handicapped parking (now DP, for Disabled Person) license plates—who could use them, where to expect the parking to be, and how to go through the process of getting them. I remember thinking it was interesting that disabled people had their own center. It was just an office, but it impressed me that some people at the school (Anthony and someone else, it turned out) had determined that disabled or handicapped people might have special needs. At that time, there was not much in the way of handicapped parking in most places, other than in front of hospitals, doctors' offices, and schools. I don't know what else the Resource Center might have offered, but it was a wakeup call for me that our needs were being addressed. I also learned that the city of Berkeley was particularly focused on disability accommodation, though this had not been true six years before at Arts and Crafts College in Oakland, with its countless stairs.

When I was in my forties, I saw that being handicapped

was similar to being a person of color in that it meant many people considered you "less than." I had not fully realized that I was part of a minority group and that there was some substantial discrimination toward us, other than that of mean school children, before then. (I say "toward" rather than "against" us because this bias is more unconscious than racism, and more similar to ageism.)

In 1980, building accessibility for disabled people, especially wheelchair users, was first implemented in Berkeley, at last. In July 1990, the Americans with Disabilities Act (ADA) was passed, largely due to the efforts of Judith Heumann and her supporters. I learned a little about its intended benefits in the summer of 1995, when I had one of my more serious falls: The handicapped parking spaces had been moved two or three lanes away from the main entrance of the store the lot served, so that one had to cross several lanes of potential traffic to get to the door. I slipped on the newly oiled paving and broke my polio kneecap. It was quite traumatic.

I later talked to an attorney about it, just wondering if there was any liability on the part of the shopping center. I was on crutches for about six weeks and worked nearly full time for each of those weeks, since I was a sole proprietor. The buck stopped with me. I had a rough time of it. Months later, as I was just beginning to heal, my attorney said, "Why yes, Francine, in fact, a few years ago the Americans with Disabilities Act (ADA) was passed, and I believe it may cover just such an incident."

The case went to mediation a year or so later. What seemed a delay turned out to be good for both parties. The mediating former judge was in a wheelchair, which looked favorable for me. I showed him my drawing of where the parking spots had been previously and where they were currently, requiring handicapped people to cross lanes of traffic. The normal people's spaces were closer and safer! It was no surprise that he got the point immediately and invited the attorneys and clients to look at how illogical the new placement was. I told him that it would mean more to me if they'd change the placement of the spaces than if they just gave me money. The case was quickly settled, and the shopping center avoided a lawsuit. The main expense for them was bringing all handicapped parking up to the ADA code. When I visited the center later, I was happy to see that every major entrance to the center had DP parking close by. I got a modest settlement, too (equal to perhaps two months' worth of my lower-middle-class income as a freelance accountant at the time), which allowed me to pay off some business loans. But for me the real triumph was that we got a dangerous condition changed to the more accessible state that it should have been in the first place.

If you should ever encounter a situation that seems it might be contrary to accessibility laws, I encourage you to at least inquire with the city or county government. They may simply not know about the problem. If they don't listen, get several people to join you in being squeaky wheels.

I can't say I like everything the ADA has done. My biggest complaint is with those bumpy yellow or black ramp covers at corners, driveways, store entrances . . . seemingly everywhere. (The bumps are legally called "truncated domes"—a big name for a little nuisance.) They are a serious trip hazard. I try to walk around them, but it's harder for me to step up on a curb than walk up a ramp, so I sometimes catch my drop foot, cane, or crutch on them. Contractors also sometimes think, *If some is good, more is better*, and install more of the domes than are required— an issue we are addressing in my own town on the city's accessibility committee.

At first, I thought the truncated domes were installed to keep wheelchairs from running away into lanes of traffic. But a polio survivor I know who lives in senior housing told me that they are for ambulatory blind people. They give the walker (or chair user) plenty of notice that they are about to enter a lane of traffic. I bow to my blind counterparts on this issue, but I wish someone would have thought this one through a little more thoroughly; I'm certain someone could have come up with a solution that was not such a trip hazard. For now, though, those domes are written into law and likely to be with us for at least a couple of decades.

I have also been annoyed to find that many DP parking spaces have been moved farther away from entrances (as at our local post office) due to interpretations of ADA requirements. There are regulations about the degree of the incline of a ramped sidewalk, for example, because wheelchairs can run away when going steeply downhill and are difficult to push up a steep incline. In order to set up for a gradual incline, the parking space has to be farther away, which often results in the user having to cross a lane of traffic to reach his or her destination. This has resulted in more former DP spaces getting turned into close regular parking for normies. The DP parking *may* be more convenient for wheelchair users, who are essentially riding—but it's also more dangerous for them, if it means they now have to navigate across a traffic lane with their less visible, low-sitting profile, and equally inconvenient for people with ambulatory difficulty who are still walking.

Some of the disability advocates who lobbied for the ADA were in wheelchairs, and I respect that they accomplished this major law change and that those on wheels now have far more access. But it is common for many people—probably contractors, especially—to think that all handicapped people are in wheelchairs, when the truth is that most of us are not. Distance is more of an issue to us than the incline of the ramp, and it is especially a problem when you have things to carry and have to cross traffic. We need parking that accommodates *every* type of disabled person—both impaired walkers and those in wheelchairs.

In the early 1990s, Richard and I went out to dinner one night in Mountain View, California. As I left and walked to my separate car at the back of the restaurant, where the DP parking spot was located, the manager approached me to ask a question: Would I prefer that the DP space be near the front door, where I'd have to cross a lane of traffic, or that it be where it was—a long walk from the door, but with a sidewalk the entire way? I really appreciated being asked and thanked him. This was the *only* time in fifty years that anyone with any influence over a public DP problem, other than the mediation judge, had ever asked for my opinion. (I *was* recently asked by a city official to sit on the accessibility committee I mentioned earlier—so that's three times in seventy years!)

That night, I told the restaurant manager that the most helpful thing would be to have one DP spot in each location available—that people who walk with assistive devices need the shortest possible distance to the front door, while people in wheelchairs, in order to be safe, need that they not be required to cross lanes of traffic.

There are still so many places that handicapped people cannot go. And that doesn't even begin to address the old stigmas that, although they are gradually falling away, still exist—prejudices such as, "Crips don't look good, so avoid hiring them." My auditing teacher in the late 1970s looked right at me in class when he said that the big eight accounting firms were very discriminatory and paid considerable attention to how you looked. You could not expect to be a person of color or to bring a brown bag lunch in those days. Women at that time could not even wear pant suits! This was an environment where the ADA countered discrimination decades later.

The *New York Times* ran an article less than a decade ago about how people with disabilities are treated by physicians here in the US. Researchers (who were MDs) called 250 doctors' offices and tried to make appointments for fictional disabled patients. Sixty-five of those offices (26 percent) refused to book an appointment, mostly because they had no adaptable or adjustable equipment, or no wheelchair access. The 185 offices (74 percent) that did book appointments also often admitted that they had no appropriate equipment, and some said they would only do parts of an examination (!?). I can imagine that this may be partly because exam tables don't usually go down low enough so that a person can transfer from a wheelchair to the table, let alone that medical offices may not have transfer slings and other similar equipment available. This is understandable—equipment is expensive—but a clinic could at least refer patients to an office that has accessibility. Less than 10 percent of those 250 offices had appropriate equipment or staff trained to assist disabled patients!

The author who reviewed this *New York Times* article, Gary Presley (author of *Seven Wheelchairs: A Life Beyond Polio*), points out that, particularly as polio survivors (and people with other disabilities), we do have to advocate for ourselves, educate physicians who probably know little or nothing about our condition, and ask for what we need. This is a theme bordering upon a motto among polio survivors, but everyone could take a cue from this article. Some communities have professional patient advocates who can be hired to manage the cases of elders' medical care.

Fans of Ayn Rand and far-right Republicans should turn their heads or close their eyes while reading this next bit: If it's a given that Republicans and Libertarians tend to think everyone should make it on their own, or that charities should provide everything for those with needs that they cannot fulfill themselves—and it does seem to be a given—you can probably see that I was more or less destined to be a Democrat. Sometimes it is necessary for the government to step in to create regulations that bar discrimination. It is for the public good that all people should at least have physical site access to schools, hospitals, apartment buildings, offices, art, libraries, shopping, and parks, not to mention a lot of other places, like hotels, veterinarians, and night clubs—and let us not leave out the all-important comedy clubs! I have found that many more and varied venues now have entrance or interior ramps to accommodate us, and some also have those small hydraulic lift elevators, which I have occasionally used. They've allowed me into more than one concert, museum, or restaurant when the stairs would have been scary or difficult for me (and, for some people, impossible).

If our culture's basic human needs of housing, food, and medical care are not met, we fall below our potential to be a kind and compassionate society. Okay, call me an idealist. But why settle for less? I don't mind paying taxes in order to facilitate these things. I believe also that only a small percentage of people abuse social welfare or medical aid. So many people out there are disabled or handicapped; let's just take care of those who cannot take care of themselves.

I may have been a fringe radical in my youth, but I don't think these ideas are radical at all. They only represent thinking on a community level.

Epilogue: Always Leave
Them Laughing

———oO◯Oo———

*L*ife lived as a cosmic joke is a lot easier than life lived as a victim, even though you may actually *be* a victim. You can start by laughing at yourself for that silly thing you did that of course was not going to work, like my wheelchair-bound friends who managed to drive themselves to the real estate office and then couldn't get out of the car to enter the business. They thought this was uproariously funny—that they hadn't thought of how they'd get into the place.

In the movie *Crip Camp*, there's a scene where a married couple, both of whom have cerebral palsy (CP), are interviewed. They met at Camp Jened. The husband relates that polio survivors are at the top of the informal hierarchy of disabled people and CPs are at the bottom because of their difference in speaking ability, a point of view I'd never considered before seeing this film. When he told his parents he was going to get married, his mother said, "I understand why you would want to marry another disabled person. But why can't you choose a 'polio'?"

While watching this scene, Richard and I looked at each other and grinned. It is not easy to be a polio survivor, as you've probably gathered from this book and will learn even more about if you read *Not a Poster Child* someday. So we thought it was pretty amusing that someone thought "a polio" was a preferred choice for a mate, or that we might be seen as the top of any hierarchy. (And for the record, again, most of us hate to be called "polios." The term with which the majority of us identify is "polio survivor.")

As Wavy Gravy (Hugh Romney, the former stockbroker who became a clown) says, "If you don't have a sense of humor, it's just not funny."

And as Forrest Gump said, "That's all I have to say about that." We've come to the end of what I wanted to share with you. My desire is that you have found something in this book that's useful, inspiring, fun, or all three. As you read this, I am likely at home or maybe an accessible vacation spot, hoping that perhaps because of something you read here, you decided to get out of the house more, or make an attempt to do a little yoga or other exercise, or to try cooking a veggie a little differently, or to tell your adult children that it's time that they helped you out a bit. And if you're one of those normie adult children, partners, or friends, perhaps you now see Mom, Dad, your spouse, or your pal in a slightly different light.

So, whaddaya think? Time to get started?

Resources for Readers

—◦◦◯◦◦—

My website and blog: https://FrancineFalk-Allen.com

www.facebook.com/FrancineFalkAllenAuthor

My previous book: Not a Poster Child: Living Well with a Disability—A Memoir. Published by She Writes Press in August 2018, it has won some awards and been listed on several best-books-of-2018 lists. Available by request at all bookstores and libraries, at www.Indibound.org, at Barnes and Noble (online and in-store), and on Amazon.

Polio and Other Disability Organizations

There are many polio organizations all over the United States and in other countries, but I'll offer just two here: PHI is the most extensive and has lists of all polio organizations worldwide, and PSNUK is a UK-based, English-speaking organization representing Europe.

- *Post-Polio Health International (PHI)*, www. post-polio.org. This is *the* polio organization. They have a great website, including many articles written by polio survivors and polio doctors. There are stories about our polio experiences, great suggestions, articles on drugs, and many links to post-polio support groups, polio doctors, organizations nearest to you, and much more. They have a quarterly newsletter to which you can subscribe. 50 Crestwood Executive Center, Suite 440, St. Louis, MO 63126-1916, info@post-polio.org.

- *Polio Survivors Network of the United Kingdom*, http://poliosurvivorsnetwork.org.uk. A good European site. Good suggestions for how to communicate with doctors so they understand that your current issues could be related to previously contracting polio and are not just "normal" symptoms of aging.

Abilities.com is an organization that (in non-COVID times) holds multiple Abilities Expos each year; these are large indoor fairs where a variety of innovations (bracing, auto adaptations, scooters) can be seen and investigated. They are held in at least the following US cities, if not more: San Jose, Los Angeles, New York, and Houston. Information about these expos and myriad other resources can be found at www.abilities.com.

About Disability, www.aboutdisability.com, is an organization started by Anthony Tusler, a lifelong disability advocate (and vibrant disabled person). A wealth of info is to be found there.

American Association of Retired Persons (AARP), https:// aarp.org, publishes a magazine and monthly bulletin with lots of info for people aged fifty and older.

American Physical Therapy Association, www.apta.org, is an online directory that can help you find a physical therapist (association member) near you. They also have a consumer website, www.choosept.com. (They're recommended by Cleveland Clinic's *Arthritis Advisor* newsletter.)

Arthritis Foundation, https://arthritis.org; information about chronic pain and how to deal with it, physically and psychologically, which is applicable to more than just the various types of arthritis.

National Council on Aging, www.ncoa.org, @NCOAging, 251 18th Street South, Suite 500, Arlington, VA 22202. This is an A-rated charity specifically addressing the needs and issues of aging Americans.

Books on Post-Polio Management
Handbook on the Late Effects of Poliomyelitis for Physicians and Survivors, edited by Frederick Maynard, MD, and Joan Headley, MS. Essential reading on polio effects. Available from https://post-polio.org.

Managing Post-Polio, by Lauro Halstead, MD. This is the authoritative book on post-polio, with explanations regarding what is happening to the polio patient thirty years or more after the initial onset and how to make your life easier. Many suggestions are good for any aging person, not just polio survivors.

More Polio- or Disability-Related Reading (plus a video)

My article "Conquering Mysterious Foot Pain," published in the PHI newsletter, can be found at www.polioplace.org/sites/default/files/files/PH28-4p1,4-5.pdf. It delineates the odyssey I went through after discovering that I had acute tendinitis and tenosynovitis in my strong foot, caused by a fallen arch and a shoe strap, and how I eventually healed this condition. There are also links within the article to the exercises that were essential to my healing. The link may say the article is in Japanese (the Japanese polio community was especially interested in the article), but it's not!

My article "The Wild Handicapper in Yosemite" (*Ability Magazine*, Feb/Mar 2016), which was adapted from the Yosemite section in this book, can be found at www.ability magazine.com/ray-romano-digital-issue/ then scroll to page 30. Also see www.polioplace.org/history/artifacts/accessible-yosemite for more on Yosemite.

The War on Microbes, PBS/Nobel Media in partnership with Kikim Media. This is a half-hour film on the eradication of diseases through immunizations in which I appear as the only polio representative interviewed, and also the only person in the film who talks about what it was like to have a communicable disease that has since been nearly eradicated through the use of vaccines. You can view it at www.vimeo.com/109047455.

"Sixtieth Anniversary for Polio Pioneers," by Karie Young-dahl, shares stories from people who participated in Jonas Salk's 1954 blinded polio vaccine trial. It can be found at https://www.historyofvaccines.org/content/blog/sixtieth-anniversary-polio-pioneers.

"When Meeting Friends with Disabilities," thirteen general rules from Easter Seals on how to treat friends with disabilities, written for children but applicable to any age: http://es.easterseals.com/site/PageServer?pagename=ntl_friends_hints.

Helpful Technologies

Dynamic Bracing Solutions, www.dynamicbracingsolutions .net. Contact for an orthotist near you. Not for everyone, but those with less severe polio effects may find this brace very helpful. BracingSolutions@aol.com.

Human Gait Institute, www.humangaitinstitute.org. Training orthotists, research of orthoses for musculo-skeletal deficits, some financial support for newer orthotic technology for those who need it. Closely connected with Dynamic Bracing. 9461 W. 37th Place, Wheat Ridge, CO 80031-5438, (303) 829-1538.

Lofstrand crutches: The best brand of these arm cuff crutches I know of is WalkEasy (www.walkeasy.com), based in Florida. They ship all over; the crutches are made in Germany and France, depending on size, so they are available in Europe as well, though probably under a different name. They come in lots of different colors, too!

TravelScoot, www.travelscoot.com. These scooters are made in Germany. I love mine: it's lightweight, comes apart, and the heaviest part weighs only about twenty-four pounds. No lift is necessary for putting it into a trunk or the back of a car. You do not take it apart for plane travel; you just remove the lithium battery and take that into the cabin, and the scooter is taken to the hold, just like a baby stroller. It is not recommended for people who have severe mental difficulty or a poor sense of balance, since it is tricky on hills with slanted paths. (800) 342-2214 in the USA; website also directs you to foreign availability.

Pride Go-Go scooters (www.pridemobility.com) are also an option, though these require either a van with a lift or a strong individual to lift the parts on the models that disassemble (the heaviest piece on the small model weighs about thirty-five pounds). These and heavier models are fine to rent, and may serve you better on rougher grassy or graveled terrain.

Disabled or Handicapped Sports
Achieve Tahoe, www.achievetahoe.org, located in Truckee, CA, administers snow and water ski and other sports for

disability challenges of all types. Originally part of Disabled Sports USA.

Disabled Sports USA, www.disabledsportsusa.org. Snow and water sports for people with disabilities, including mental disabilities.

National Ability Center, www.discovernac.org. Programs for the differently abled in many sports.

Achieve Tahoe Adaptive Programs, www.achievetahoe.org, Alpine Meadows, South Lake Tahoe, CA. Snow ski instruction for the ability-challenged. Other adaptive ski schools are available in the Tahoe area at Squaw Valley and Heavenly Valley; this is the original location with the instructors who helped set up the other adaptive programs.

Disabled, Physically Challenged, or Handicapped Travel

Guides and Trip Planning

Lonely Planet accessible travel guides, https://shop.lonely planet.com/products/accessible-travel-online-resources -2019. These are free and downloadable, printed guides. There will not be an update beyond 2019, because Martin Heng, who wrote the guides, retired from Lonely Planet. Lonely Planet also has a helpful forum for challenged travelers, located at www.lonelyplanet.com/thorntree/ forums/welcome. From there, search "travelers with disabilities."

The Rough Guide (published in New York, London, and Delhi) and Lonely Planet (published in Oakland, London, and Melbourne) are my overall favorite travel guides for just about any destination. While these are not specifically written for handicapped travel, they often describe the difficulty of a particular walking route and, importantly, exactly how long it is, as well as whether there is an elevator where you want to go. They also sometimes indicate wheelchair accessibility. I have also used the AAA guides (Automobile Association of America).

I use *TripAdvisor* (www.tripadvisor.com) frequently to search hotels, though once I find lodging that seems well located, has a pool, and doesn't require me to use stairs, I follow up by calling to see if there is accessibility for the pool, the front door, and whatever else I need in order to be comfortable there. TripAdvisor reviews tend to be reliable, and I have reviewed about one hundred hotels myself on that site. Rarely does anyone address disability issues, so I always note whether there are accessibility problems (even if I can manage but a wheelchair user would have difficulty).

Other Travel Websites
Accessible Cruise Planners—worldwide destinations. My info says, "Ask for Steve." (800) 801-9002.

Access Tours, www.accesstours.org, offers accessible package tours of National Parks and other areas in the western states. (800) 929-4811.

Accessible Journeys, www.accessiblejourneys.com, is dedicated to travel for people in wheelchairs and their companions.

Angloinfo "People with Disabilities" page, www.angloinfo.com/how-to/france/healthcare/people-with-disabilities. Disability info for English-speaking travelers in Paris, France.

MyHandicap, www.myhandicap.com. A European site; not a lot of info, but a start.

National Park Service "Accessibility" page, www.nps.gov/accessibility.htm. Here you can download the National Park Service's access guide for visitors and potential employees. I download this guide when I go to Yosemite to update myself on their latest wooden and paved pathways and options.

No Limits Foundation, www.nolimitsfoundation.org, provides a camping experience to children who have lost a limb. They also partner with Yosemite National Park to bring wheelchair access there.

Sage Travelling, www.sagetraveling.com "The European Disabled Travel Experts." Hotels, tours, group travel, and access guides for all major European cities and many more. Recommended by Rick Steves' Europe.

VacationsToGo "Travelers with Special Needs" page, www.vacationstogo.com/special_needs_cruises.cfm. Information about the special-needs facilities, amenities, and services provided by a number of cruise companies.

Yosemite Conservancy "No Limits: Yosemite Adventures for Wheelchair Users—2017" page, https://yosemite.org/projects/no-limits-yosemite-adventures-for-wheelchair-users-2017. A program partnering with the No Limits Foundation to provide greater access to more locations within Yosemite National Park for adult and youth wheelchair users, with adaptive outdoor recreation assistants. (There may be a later year update, so try Googling "No Limits: Yosemite" if a specific year doesn't bring up the page.)

Buying Mis-Mated Shoes

National Odd Shoe Exchange, www.oddshoe.org, located in Chandler, AZ, accepts new mis-mated shoes as charitable donations and also matches people with mis-mated shoes, though I have not been successful in determining how to trade shoes in the last several decades. I just donate my mis-mates and take a tax deduction.

Nordstrom, www.nordstrom.com. You buy the two different-sized pairs and then ship back the mis-mates (with an explanatory letter and request for refund), and they give you a credit card refund for the price of the less expensive pair. When purchasing two pairs in a store for one set of feet, they will only charge for the more expensive pair.

Zappos, www.zappos.com. They do not split pairs, but this is the easiest way I have found of buying shoes: just buy two pairs and donate the leftovers. They also provide free shipping coming and going.

Yoga DVDs

"Arthritis-Friendly Yoga," Arthritis Foundation, DVD available from www.arthritis.org, 2015.

"Easy Yoga for Arthritis," DVD available from www.shop pbs.org. They also offer other helpful DVDs that are listed in their catalog under "Survival Guide for Pain-Free Living."

(Do look online for other books and DVDs on chair or bed yoga. The bed yoga DVD I have is out of print.)

Charities Benefiting Indian Orphans

SOS Children's Villages, www.sos-usa.org. Places orphans in a stable home for the rest of their lives. Many go on to college and do relevant social work to "pay back" the assistance they received.

Friends of Ramana's Garden, www.friendsramanasgarden. org. US organization supporting Ramana's Garden in India; provides healthcare for children living in extreme poverty and their families.

The Hope Project, www.childrensashramfund.org. Sufi organization that provides food, schooling, and vocational training for orphans.

Bibliography and
Suggested Reading

----∘○◯○∘----

Baum, Glenda. *Aquarobics, the Training Manual*. Philadelphia: W.B. Saunders, 1998.

Bhandari, Neena. "India Needs to Focus on Its Polio Survivors." *Post-Polio Health* 31:2 (2015).

Bishop, Jack. *Vegetables Every Day*. New York: Harper Collins, 2001.

Bogardus, Meghan. "You've Seen Them Care, Now Show You Care About Them." *AARP The Magazine*, October/November 2015.

Burgess, Kaya. "Brush Teeth Three Times a Day for a Healthier Heart." *The Times* (London, UK), December 2, 2019.

Butler, David, MAppSc, and Lorimer Moseley, PhD. *Explain Pain*. Adelaide, Australia: Noigroup Publications, 2003.

Crocker, Ann. "What to Eat: Revisiting the Basics." *Post-Polio Health* 32:2 (2016).

Daggett, Richard. "Polio Facts." *Sacramento Post-Polio Support Group Newsletter*, April 2009.

Dass, Ram. *Be Here Now.* San Cristobal, NM: Lama Foundation, 1971.

Doucleff, Michaeleen. "Why Bill Gates Thinks Ending Polio Is Worth It." *Post-Polio Health International Newsletter*, May 2013.

The Economist. "Democracy in America." October 29, 2009.

Erickson, Mandy. "Alcoholics Anonymous most effective path to alcohol abstinence." *Stanford Medicine News Center*, March 2020.

Haiken, Melanie. "A New Leaf." *Marin Magazine*, April 2017.

Halstead, Lauro, MD. *Managing Post-Polio: A Guide to Living Well with Post-Polio Syndrome.* Arlington: ABI Professional Publications, 1998/2005.

Harvard Medical School. *Core Exercises.* Boston: Harvard Health Publications, 2013.

Harvard Medical School. *Knees and Hips* Boston: Harvard Health Publications, 2015.

Harvard Medical School. *Stretching*. Boston: Harvard Health Publications, 2012.

Harvard Women's Health Watch. "Behavioral activation therapy effectively treats depression, study finds." October 2016.

Harvard Women's Health Watch. "Can supplements help boost your immune system?" January 2020.

Harvard Women's Health Watch. "Getting a start on growing stronger." July 2017.

Harvard Women's Health Watch. "Music to your brain." September 2020.

Harvard Women's Health Watch. "Treating pain with your brain." September 2016. www.health.harvard.edu/mind-and-mood/treating-pain-with-your-brain.

Headley, Joan L., MS, and Frederick M. Maynard, MD, with Stephanie T. Machell, PsyD, and Holly H. Wise, PT, PhD. *Post-Polio Health Care Considerations for Families & Friends*. St. Louis, MO: Post-Polio Health International, 2011, www.post-polio.org.

Heumann, Judith. *Being Heumann: An Unrepentant Memoir of a Disability Rights Advocate*. Boston: Beacon Press, 2020.

Huckert, Greg. "Integral Orthotics and Prosthetics." A talk given at Sacramento Post-Polio Support Group, May 3, 2014 (published as notes in their newsletter, September 2014).

Hurme, Sally Balch, and Lawrence A. Frolik. *ABA/AARP Wise Moves: Checklist for Where to Live, What to Consider, and Whether to Stay or Go.* Chicago, IL: American Bar Association, March 7, 2020.

Junger, Sebastian. "The Bonds of Battle—The Never-Ending War." *Vanity Fair,* June 2015.

Kabat, Herman, MD, and Miland E. Knapp, MD. "The Use of Prostigmine in the Treatment of Poliomyelitis." *Journal of the American Medical Association*, August 7, 1943.

LaMotte, Sanddee. "Your hatred of heart-healthy veggies could be genetic." CNN.com, November 14, 2019.

Li, Ying. "Mu Mengjie—The Power of a Teacher's Love." *Ability* (Huntington Beach, CA), 2015.

Linden, David. "Fingertips To Hair Follicles: Why 'Touch' Triggers Pleasure And Pain." *Fresh Air*, February 3, 2015.

Machell, Stephanie T., PsyD. "Promoting Positive Solutions." *Post-Polio Health* 32:2 (2016).

Maynard, Frederick, MD, and Joan Headley, MS. *Handbook on the Late Effects of Poliomyelitis for Physicians and Survivors*. St. Louis: Gazette International Networking Institute, 1999. Available from www.post-polio.org.

McNeil Jr., Donald G. "Polio's Return After Near Eradication Prompts a Global Health Warning." *The New York Times*, May 5, 2014. www.nytimes.com/2014/05/06/health/world-health-organization-polio-health-emergency.html.

Merill, Michele Cohen. "Finding Her Light Within—Yoga Helped Eugenia Esquivel Cope with RA." *Arthritis Today*, The Arthritis Foundation, Winter, 2019–2020.

Mitchell, Paulette. *The 15-Minute Gourmet: Chicken*. Foster City, CA: IDG Books Worldwide, Inc., 1999.

Oshinsky, David M. *Polio: An American Story*. New York: Oxford University Press, 2005.

Parker, Amy. "Growing Up Unvaccinated." *Slate*, January 6, 2014. https://slate.com/human-interest/2014/01/growing-up-unvaccinated-a-healthy-lifestyle-couldnt-prevent-many-childhood-illnesses.html.

Perry, Cat. "Supplement Safety." *Arthritis Today*, The Arthritis Foundation. Winter, 2019–2020.

Presley, Gary. "You Can't Always Blame Other People." May 29, 2013. www.polioalberta.ca/wp-content/uploads/2018/09/Q1_2017.pdf and scroll to page 11.

Roth, Philip. *Nemesis*. New York: Houghton Mifflin Harcourt, 2010.

Schmitt, Rick. "The Stranger in Your Home." *AARP Bulletin*, March 2015.

Schroeder, Stephen M., DPM. "Triple Arthrodesis." *Medscape*, August 16, 2011. https://emedicine.medscape.com/article/1234042-overview.

Scrase, Richard. "Sixty years of the polio 'miracle' vaccine." *Understanding Animal Research*, April 13, 2015. http://www.understandinganimalresearch.org.uk/news/video-of-the-week/sixty-years-of-the-polio-miracle-vaccine.

Sedaker, Cheryl. *365 Ways to Cook Chicken*. New York: Harper & Row, 1986.

Seltzer, Beverly. *The Lady and the Lingcod*. Victoria, BC: Trafford Publishing, 2003.

Shapiro, Joseph P. *No Pity: People with Disabilities Forging a New Civil Rights Movement*. New York: Random House, 1993.

Shreve, Susan Richards. *Warm Springs*. New York: Mariner Books, 2007.

The Week. "Bionic breakthrough." March 13, 2015.

The Week. "Boring but important—The globe goes gray." April 8, 2016.

The Week. "Hate broccoli? Blame your genes." Valerie Duffy, University of Connecticut, CNN.com, November 29, 2019.

The Week. "Life-hacking the new year." January 17, 2020.

The Week. "Some of the things they said were good for us . . ." December 27, 2019/January 10, 2020.

The Week. "The future of artificial limbs." March 22, 2014. http://theweek.com/articles/448972/future-artificial -limbs.

Thompson, Dennis. "The Salk Polio Vaccine: A Medical Miracle Turns 60." *HealthDay*, December 1, 2014. https://consumer.healthday.com/infectious-disease -information-21/misc-infections-news-411/the-salk- polio-vaccine-a-medical-miracle-turns-60-691863.html.

UCLA Health. "The opioid epidemic and seniors." *Healthy Years* 14:5 (May 2016).

UCLA Health. "A brief history of the prescription opioid epidemic." *Healthy Years* 14:5 (May 2016).

Verville, Richard. *War, Politics, and Philanthropy: The History of Rehabilitation Medicine*. Lanham, MD: University Press of America, 2009.

Wang, Penelope. "How to Talk to Your Parents about Moving Out of Their Big Beautiful House." Money.com, November 18, 2016.

Watkins, Robert G., Bill Buhler, and Patricia Loverock. *The Water Workout Recovery Program: Safe and Painless Exercises for Treating Back Pain, Muscle Tears, Tendinitis, Sports Injuries, and More.* Chicago: Contemporary Books, 1988.

Weisberg, Joseph, PT, PhD, and Heidi Shink. *Three Minutes to a Pain-Free Life.* New York: Atria Books/Simon and Schuster, 2005.

Wilson, Daniel J. *Polio (Biographies of Disease).* Santa Barbara, CA: Greenwood Press, 2009.

Winters, Catherine. "When Words Hurt." *Arthritis Today*, March/April 2016.

Zimmerman, Mike. "Who Gets Sick and Why." *AARP Bulletin*, May 2020.

Please see the Bibliography section of *Not a Poster Child: Living Well with a Disability—A Memoir* for more reading on polio and vaccine-preventable diseases.

Acknowledgments

⸻◦○○◦⸻

Thank you to the people who encouraged me to keep the parts of my first book that were actually more self-help than memoir, which were the hatchlings for this big bird of a book—especially Shirley Klock, who thought this might be a useful tome. Gratitude and props to my writing group, Just Write Marin County, especially Aline O'Brien, Maryan Karwan, Marcia Naomi Berger (thanks for doing a beta read), Jacqueline Bradley, Ed Janne, and Nancy Harris. These friends have listened to me squawk, as well as trill when I met with success, and given me a lot of seeds to follow along my path to completion. On a more personal level, this is also true of my close friends in my two women's groups, who listen to me about my writing, my nest, my love bird, and so much more.

Thanks to Emmy Lou Noble, my water-exercise teacher, who not only taught me the ducky set that has served me for over twenty years but also scrambled to get me copies of illustrations and the names of the best water exercise books. Thanks to Martin Heng for finding the revised site address for the vital Lonely Planet accessible travel guide. And thanks to the venerable health advocates Kathryn Johnson and Judith Heumann, and also to Mary Plouffe, Ph.D, for doing read-throughs.

Thanks to the flock of people who thought *The Wild Handicapper* would be a great main title, and also the few who pointed out that it sounded like a golf book. (Who knew? Not me. Although I did know that the term "birdie" had something to do with the game.) Big time thanks to Elke Barter, inspired graphic designer, for a cover I love, after we changed the title to *No Spring Chicken*. She read my writing and somehow immediately knew what kind of image and colors I would crow about.

Thanks to my She Writes Press author friends, especially Betsy Fasbinder, Amy M. Peele, Susan Burrowes, Vanya Erickson, Nina G, Bonnie Monte, Cindy Rasicot, Mary Plouffe, Linda Gartz, Stephanie Raffelock, Kathryn Taylor, and Jodi Wright. And I'm sure there are some gulls I am forgetting to mention. All of you have given me great tips, feedback, opportunities, or encouragement—or just shared your own experience in a way that lifted my wings and let me soar.

Krissa Lagos, my able editor, sifts through my chicken scratchings (well, on the computer, let's be honest) and makes them something more cohesive, so they look like they could fly instead of resembling a bird's nest that fell out of a tree—a nice one, yes, but still in need of repair. Thank you for your patience and kind and reliable craftsmanship, Krissa!

Thanks to Chris Dumas for his proofreading and some style suggestions, half of which I agreed with, and to Megan Hannum for her meticulous final proofing.

Thanks to She Writes Press for believing in me and what I have to say, and for leading me through the thicket and preening me—most especially Brooke Warner, Lauren Wise, and Shannon Green.

And always, at the end of the day, when I fly away home to my warm nest, all my love and gratitude to Richard Falk for your support in all ways. I may be a Wild Handicapper, but I know where to roost.

About the Author

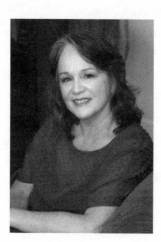

*F*rancine Falk-Allen was born in Los Angeles and has lived nearly all of her life in Northern California. A former art major with a BA in managerial accounting who ran her own business for thirty-three years, she has always craved creative outlets. This has taken the form of singing and recording with various groups, painting, and writing songs, poetry, and essays, some of which have been published. Falk-Allen facilitates Polio Survivors of Marin County and Just Write Marin County (a Meetup writing group), and is a volunteer member of the San Rafael City ADA Accessibility Committee. Her first book, *Not a Poster Child: Living Well with a Disability: A Memoir* has been included on several national outlets' lists of best books of 2018, including *Kirkus Reviews*, BuzzFeed, and PopSugar, and received a gold medal from Living Now Book Awards for Inspiring Memoir – Female and a silver medal from Sarton Women's Book Awards for memoir. She was also named one of "25 Women Making a Difference in 2019" by *Conversations Magazine*. She loves the outdoors, gardening, pool exercise, her sweet, peculiar old cat, spending time with her husband and good friends, strong British tea, and a little champagne now and then. Francine lives in San Rafael, California.

SELECTED TITLES FROM SHE WRITES PRESS

She Writes Press is an independent publishing
ompany founded to serve women writers everywhere.
Visit us at www.shewritespress.com.

Not a Poster Child: Living Well with a Disability—A Memoir by
Francine Falk-Allen. $16.95, 978-1631523915. Francine Falk-Allen
was only three years old when she contracted polio and temporarily
lost the ability to stand and walk. Here, she tells the story of how
a toddler learned grown-up lessons too soon; a schoolgirl tried her
best to be a "normie," on into young adulthood; and a woman finally
found her balance, physically and spiritually.

Role Reversal: How to Take Care of Yourself and Your Aging Parents
by Iris Waichler. $16.95, 978-1-63152-091-4. A comprehensive
guide for the 45 million people currently taking care of family
members who need assistance because of health-related problems.

A Leg to Stand On: An Amputee's Walk into Motherhood by Colleen
Haggerty. $16.95, 978-1-63152-923-8. Haggerty's candid story of
how she overcame the pain of losing a leg at seventeen—and of
terminating two pregnancies as a young woman—and went on to
become a mother, despite her fears.

Green Nails and Other Acts of Rebellion: Life After Loss by Elaine
Soloway. $16.95, 978-1-63152-919-1. An honest, often humorous
account of the joys and pains of caregiving for a loved one with a
debilitating illness.

Not by Accident: Reconstructing a Careless Life by Samantha Dunn.
$16.95, 978-1-63152-832-3. After suffering a nearly fatal riding
accident, lifelong klutz Samantha Dunn felt compelled to examine
just what it was inside herself—and other people—that invited
carelessness and injury.